Trust me I am ~~NOT~~ a Doctor!

A.J. Mueller

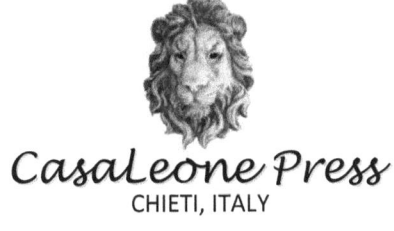

CHIETI, ITALY

Copyright © 2018 A.J. Mueller

All rights reserved. No part of this book may be reproduced, stored in a retrieval system or transmitted in any form or by any means without the prior written approval of A.J. Mueller except by a reviewer who may quote brief passages in a review to be printed in a newspaper, magazine or journal.

ISBN: 978-0-9970118-0-7
Published in the USA by CasaLeone Press

To my wonderful wife Marsha for putting up with me not only as I was writing this book but for tolerating me and my 'creativity' during our whole life together.

To my awesome children Andrew, Claudine, Danielle, Darren, Gary and Nikki as well as my sisters Carol, Debbie, Jackie, Mary Ellen and the memories of Margie, brother George,
Mom and Dad.

THIS BOOK IS A REFLECTION OF ONLY MY PERSONAL THOUGHTS. ANY MENTION OR SUGGESTION OF OTHERS WHO WERE SUPPORTIVE OF ME AND MY EFFORTS IN THE PAST DOES NOT MEAN THAT THEY SUPPORT MY PRESENT VIEWS AND ASSERTIONS CONTAINED IN THIS BOOK.

SPECIAL DEDICATION

To My sister Margaret Mueller-Ottesen, Dominic Lumbruno, the Honorable Judge Joseph Padawer and all others who suffered unnecessarily before death at the hands of those medical professionals who dismissed or misused the available modern technologies on those who placed their ultimate trust in their hands. May they find eternal piece and comfort in the hands of their creator.

Who commits the most egregious crime; a criminal who unintentionally kills someone with a weapon during the commission of a crime, or a doctor who willingly and knowingly inflicts pain and suffering on a dying patient through the over-utilization of modern technologies and procedures for the sole purpose of extending life for financial gain?

This book is also dedicated to all of those cardiologists, radiologists, researchers, physicists and other medical professionals that allowed me into their world and taught me what I needed to know to assist in the fulfillment of our mutual goals.

A very, very special thanks goes out to all of the cardiologists, family practitioners and radiologists with whom I worked and who were the early adopters of cardiovascular computed tomography for calcium screening as well as CVCT angiography. It was an honor and a pleasure to have worked with all of you.

I truly believe that the patients of all of these early adapters of CVCT owe their doctors a great debt of gratitude for placing their health and welfare ahead of all else, including profits, in their practices.

CONTENTS

1	Introduction to my 'Mission'	Pg 12
2	Common Sense Cardiology?	Pg 21
3	Voodoo Medicine?	Pg 31
4	Traditional (Non-Voodoo) Medicine?	Pg 38
5	May the (magnetic) force be with you	Pg 44
6	The Kidneys and Urolithiasis (Froggy Litho)	Pg 51
7	Common Sense and Disease Prevention	Pg 63
8	Wanes, Wessels, Pluck and where the hell is Perry Ferrel?	Pg 71
	SECTION TWO – The Human Anatomy	Pg 84
9	The Human Heart	Pg 85
10	The Human Blood	Pg 88
11	The Human Liver	Pg 90
12	The Human Kidneys	Pg 92
13	The Human Skin	Pg 94
14	The Human Eye	Pg 97
15	The Human Throat	Pg 100
16	The Human Ear	Pg 103
	ABOUT THE AUTHOR	Pg 106

Perhaps the greatest dichotomy in life is that you really do not know your 'outer limits' until you actually surpass them.

Forward

I first met Mr. Mueller while working in Santa Monica California as a cardiologist and early adopter of non-invasive coronary artery imaging. As a clinician, I found a parallel excitement in this burgeoning field with Mr. Mueller, who was at that time a technical consultant to Siemens Medical Systems. We have worked together since that time as friends and as colleagues.

Mr. Mueller's knowledge base draws on over 20 years of business and engineering experience in the technical and medical elements of computed tomographic imaging: initially with non-contrast CT, followed my contrast enhanced CT. He has had a vision of using this technology and the evolving tools that accompany it to "do the right thing for patients": that is, to use it to guide the discovery and treatment of occult coronary artery disease for superior patient outcomes. This has been his unfailing mantra, and he has achieved a comprehensive understanding of the economic and clinical issues that surround Cardiac Computed tomography. I often speak with Mr. Mueller and have to remind myself that he is an engineer and a businessman, not a physician.

His technical and scientific grasp of the physics and engineering of X-radiation, CT image creation, network systems and visualization are excellent. More importantly, his grasp of the clinical meaning of "value" and "accuracy" in the changing patient management scenarios we are going through in this country is ideologically sound. As such I believe Mr. Mueller is particularly able to frame the argument of the need to control diagnostic testing from its current run away course.

We share the view that CTA and Calcium scoring have the potential to guide patient care in ways that are currently only beginning.

Finally, Mr. Mueller has been instrumental in the progress that CTA has experienced. He enjoys close professional and personal relationships with many of the pioneers and thought leaders in the SCAI and the SCCT. He brings ideas and people together ultimately for the advantage of patient care. He is a fine man and a distinguished colleague.

CARTER NEWTON MD FACC
ASSISTANT PROFESSOR OF RADIOLOGY AND ASSISTANT CLINICAL PROFESSOR OF CARDIOLOGY
UNIVERSITY OF ARIZONA, COLLEGE OF MEDICINE

I have known Mr. Mueller for many years. We have worked closely on past ventures as well as potential future projects which focus on innovative utilization of emerging technologies.

Mr. Mueller's role has been, and continues to be, an expert in targeting these technologies. He has been instrumental in the development of strategies promoting highly innovative and efficient use of high technology resources within managed care.

To accomplish this he has an effective and highly unique approach: complete immersion in the targeted technology until, by applying his broad repertoire of analytical and technical skills, he masters the mechanics, use, and value of the technology.

Of special importance to me as a managed care medical director is the latter. Mr. Mueller has the unique ability to recognize new and better uses for state of the art technology, innovative in scope and value.

[signature]

JOSEPH G COCKE, MD
MEDICAL DIRECTOR
BLUE CROSS BLUE SHIELD OF FLORIDA

Mr. Mueller has enjoyed a professional relationship with Siemens Medical Systems, Inc. and me for decades. Siemens has worked with Mr. Mueller only on cutting edge, emerging technology projects. Several years ago Mr. Mueller purchased, paid for, and installed a Siemens lithotripter when waterless lithotripsy was the newest technology and his efforts greatly expanded the clinical application and more importantly, managed care acceptance of Optimized-Pressure lithotripsy.

For the past several years, since introducing A.J. to Electron Beam Technology Ultrafast CT, he has become one of the foremost authorities on the technology in the world.

After numerous visits to Siemens global investigational sites and direct involvement with the Imatron factory in South San Francisco his knowledge and clinical vision for this technology has been further enhanced. He truly understands this technology and its practical usage as it applies to the managed care communities.

We at Siemens eagerly anticipate Mr. Mueller's continuing involvement with us regarding this valuable technology and the additional benefits to be derived from a comprehensive coronary artery screening program being established by him in Florida.

Having spent my entire career with Siemens, watching Mr. Mueller once again develop this program to its present level, I wholeheartedly endorse A.J.'s vision for this technology in general, and for Mr. Mueller in particular.

Both I and Siemens look forward to his efforts into the future.

Sincerely
Siemens Medical Systems, Inc.

PAT VARAN,
CARDIOVASCULAR ACCOUNTS MANAGER

THE AUTHORS OF THESE ENDORSEMENTS AND THE INSTITUTIONS THAT THEY REPRESENT DO NOT NECESSARILY SHARE IN THE PERSONAL THOUGHTS AND SOMEWHAT DELICATE SUPPOSITIONS ASSERTED BY ME IN THIS BOOK!

CHAPTER ONE

"Stupidity lives within you forever; ignorance, however, can be rendered a much shorter–term problem."

Every story should have a beginning, an end and something riveting, hopefully inspiring, educational, motivating and entertaining that separates the two. In many stories, such as this one, it is often difficult to determine a definite beginning, and in some cases, such as this one, the end, thank God, is yet to be determined.

This book is an absolute testament to the fact that one person can indeed make a difference even in a most complex area of society such as medicine and the distribution of same through the even more intricate areas of the modern-day health care delivery system.

Over the last four decades I have been contracted by many Medical Technology firms, mainly Siemens Medical of Germany, to assist in the development of strategies for the validation, introduction and systemic integration of many emerging technologies into the mainstream American health care delivery system. These included Nuclear Magnetic Resonance (now known as the more patient-friendly Magnetic Resonance Imaging) for enhanced visualization of deep internal organs; Optimized-Pressure Extracorporeal Shockwave Lithotripsy (ESWL) for treatment and management of Urolithiasis, Vertebral Axial Decompression (VaxD) for the relief of back disorders and Cardiovascular Computed Tomography (CVCT) for the detection, identification and quantification of Coronary Artery Disease (CAD) and Peripheral Vessel Disease (PVD).

Putting money where my mouth was over that same period of time I have personally owned and operated multiple MRI imaging centers, an Optimized-Pressure Lithotripsy center which was the first ever to be contracted by Blue Cross & Blue Shield and two Cardiovascular Imaging centers which were also among the first to be contracted by BC & BS for Cardiovascular studies in the United States. I have also been designated by a number of States including Texas (<u>State of Texas certificate # TXC 0001205</u>) as an 'expert' in the utilization of Cardiovascular CT for the detection, management and treatment of Cardiovascular Disease.

I have made Cardiovascular Disease Management presentations at Stanford University, Harvard Med School and the University of Munich Med Center. I have consulted with and lectured to thousands of cardiologists in the United States, England, Germany, Italy, France, Austria, Switzerland, Puerto Rico, Canada, Dubai, Bahrain, Qatar, Abu Dhabi and Yemen. I have worked closely with many groups in the States, Europe and the United Arab Emirates in the development of local and regional Heart Attack Prevention programs, CVCT centers as well as in the development of standardized training programs and protocols for both cardiologists and physicians in the proper utilization of CVCT.

I have done this with the open admission, up front and center, that I am not a cardiologist nor am I a physician; I am not even a PHD! To this day I remain somewhat dumbfounded that, out of all of the people accessible to Siemens across the globe, I was chosen to spearhead the development and implementation of strategies for the introduction and integration of Cardiovascular CT into the United States health care marketplace. There is one other significant fact that makes my personal positive impact in the world of cardiology even more unbelievable but also highly inspirational; I never graduated High School; in fact I never finished grade 11. It was not because I lacked the mental faculties to do so; I was always in the top of my class. It was the unfortunate result of my family falling victim to a financial disaster which, at least in my mind at that time, took priority and dictated that I do all in my power to help my siblings keep my Mother and the family afloat. I felt that I had no choice, I simply had to go to work, full-time, which I did.

I can say without any reservation that I was chosen for this position by the executives of Siemens because I was without question the most prepared person for the position and the most capable of doing what had to be done. The Siemens executives did not even inquire about my educational background; I believe that they just assumed that I was a doctor as a result of my acceptance by the cardiology community and my ability to converse effectively on the clinical level with the cardiologists!

In all honesty; I was in fact more than up to the task. I had taken years and years to not only access the best research physicians and physicists but to have them personally instill their years and years of knowledge and experience directly into my brain. I became extremely well educated and fully conversant in all pertinent areas of cardiology and CT technology. As a result I quickly acquired a very unique understanding of the underlying principles of CT technology, the structure and functionality of the Heart, the biomechanical processes of Coronary Artery Disease and how CVCT could positively affect patient outcomes in the practice of cardiology.

This most unique combination of technical and medical knowledge, coupled with my ability and ease in effectively dealing with complex medical issues found me up front and center stage, literally, in educating the cardiology community in the scientific and clinical value of the technology as well as the proper protocols and methods for effective utilization of CVCT in their practices. Over a very few years with the company I became the Director of Cardiology Segment Development for Siemens Global Solutions out of Germany

My stated personal mission since 1978 has been 'to provide superior patient outcomes through the proper utilization of superior technologies' so this foray into the world of Cardiology was the perfect fit. I am proud to have been a pioneer in all of the areas of medicine in which I got involved. I am especially proud to have had such positive impact on patient's lives resulting from enhanced clinical outcomes through the subsequent programmed utilization of the many emerging technologies that I helped advance; especially in the cardiovascular arena.

If you wish to make a significant change in any complex environment the very first thing that you must do is take the 'blinders' off and look beyond your own mental fences, other barricades and self-imposed obstacles. There are opportunities galore for consequential change out there; you just have to find the proper path to go down to strategically plant the seeds for your own 'mission'.

Don't be mistaken; forcing meaningful change is not an easy task by any stretch of the imagination, however, it can definitely be done if one is fully prepared with targeted education, factual knowledge of the subjects at hand and is tastefully persistent. You must also be thick-skinned, personally organized and willing to tactfully take a stand at whatever level necessary to secure the essential audience who can enthusiastically digest, accept and, even more importantly, actually advance the mental paradigm shift required to affect meaningful change.

Sometimes it actually requires thoughtful but forceful unrelenting psychological incursions to get the attention of those at the helm. A good friend and health care business mentor extraordinaire, Tim Attebery, used to refer to me as the 'hornet in the car' forcing everyone to put on the mental brakes and really listen to what I was saying.

It is no secret that there are growing numbers of Americans who have serious misgivings regarding our present health care system ranging from the motives and direction from the President of the United States, State and Federal government legislators and agencies, insurance company executives, right down to questions regarding the moral principles guiding those on the frontlines of the health care battle; the doctors that dole out medical care. The physicians are increasingly in the bull's eye of the target and, unfortunately for the general public, deservingly so resulting from their evolving business policies that strategically hand out their health care in a way that is anything but personal and compassionate.

This book is in no way an attempt to engage in any type of process that could somehow render the present system of health care delivery invalid, nor am I attempting to fan the flames of an already skeptical, but also somewhat uneducated, public. I just want to add a tad more fuel to the mounting suspicions and public distrust of those directly involved in the health care delivery system; fuel that may further engage and encourage those who can effect even more meaningful change to do so.

My primary objective in writing this book is to offer a fresh, different and unique perspective of medicine and today's unwieldy health care delivery system together with special thoughts on the various personal and professional responsibilities that should be integral to the entire process. This rather exclusive viewpoint you will find is not based upon the present-day system of patient assessment founded in antiquated, questionable speculation itself based upon even more dubious assumptions and teachings from centuries past. The perspective of this book is based upon good old common sense, pertinent up-to-date information and knowledge mixed in with relevant historical data. All of this must be viewed in the context of a specific personal pseudo-research project based upon one man's travel from irresponsible youth to rather vigorous geriatrics; my journey. I have made it to 70 plus years of age while defying the odds of death for decades, at least according to many, many physicians and clinical experts who were, for assorted reasons, called on to care for me and occasionally piece me back together over those decades.

From early in my teenage years I have been given numerous warnings of imminent death from cancer, heart disease and hyper-elevated blood pressure yet here I am today still going strong! Why? Because of luck, a healthy dose of skepticism, an innate ability to filter out reality from hype, a fear of professional incompetence and, above all, the increasingly elusive good old common sense.

Those who know me recognize me as more than just a bit of a skeptic; I could easily be the poster child for skepticism. I truly am a cynic's cynic, sort of like Clark Gable being an actor's actor. I suspect that from my very first breath this trait had a stronghold on my brain. Fortunately, at least for me, is the fact that I was also bestowed at birth with a great dose of the aforementioned common sense. From as far back as I can recall I took very few details as factual until I had a chance to let my common sense mentally regurgitate and 'check them out' for myself. Like a judge my brain would then render a verdict for me to use on the weight of the evidence. I openly confess to being a verifiable misanthropist, not in a negative way as one would think but in a way that would allow the truth of the issues to filter through my brain and guide me in the proper direction; for good or bad, but at least I would be dealing in reality. I refer to my over abundance of skepticism as sort of having my own personal mental 'jury' with me, full-time, and me being the judge. And unlike our present somewhat flawed, intentionally convoluted judicial system I, as the judge, have the final say; period, full stop! In direct contrast to our present legal system I absolutely refuse to put the final decision on exactly how I will handle so called factual information in the hands of those who know little or nothing of how my brain actually works and more importantly, how it guides me through my life. Question one; who else knows better than you how you operate? Answer; no-one; you do! Common sense and constructive skepticism guides my existence and has allowed me to avoid many, many pitfalls in life and many, many more in my career; the publication of this book being an obvious exception for I suspect that this will not help at all when it comes to my standing within the medical community.

My unbridled lack of assurance in what I am being told, even by experts and even when backed up by, according to the professional provider, apparently valid research, presents its own set of challenges as I try to navigate the twisty pathways of life. Many, I am sure, may refer to my distinguishing doubtful psychological attribute as a plain old mental defect. Cerebral programming such as mine can be challenging to say the least, however, it presents an even greater and more troublesome challenge when attempting to function at the higher clinical management levels of the medical community. This is especially true when it comes to the 'inner sanctum' of the cardiovascular services sector of the health care delivery system. To add even more challenge, as if it were needed, is when an individual attempts to positively impact cardiovascular clinical outcomes when one is not a cardiologist. That would be me, the very vocal non-cardiologist cardiovascular disease management specialist. There are many cardiovascular professionals out there who dislike me not for what I say and do but simply because only am I not a cardiologist; little do they know I am not even a physician! I am just a common sense guy with a reasonable level of intelligence, knowledge, good communication skills and an innate ability to quickly determine right from wrong and good from bad.

My somewhat suspicious brain has partnered well with my common sense. Those two personal attributes, when working in concert, dish out wholesome intellectual distrust of most relative claims, disguised as the more socially acceptable cynicism. This, working in partnership with good old common sense, has given me the ability to mentally view things from a different perspective than most.

This permits me to perceive things that others either did not see, or worse yet, refused to acknowledge. My skeptical-based common sense has permitted me to get to, and stay, 'cutting edge' as far as medical diagnostic and therapeutic technologies are concerned.

This 'cutting edge' mentality allows me to achieve an envious position of determining the efficacy and potential integration of technologies far ahead of most of the other individuals; individuals who are simply fact-based. My ability to quickly ferret out the 'real deal' has brought about huge clinical and lifestyle benefits for all who have found themselves, for whatever reasons, placed directly or indirectly in my more than capable hands for their clinical wellbeing.

Let's take a couple of steps forward and look at a few hypothetical scenarios; situations that in reality take place thousands of times each and every day in this country.

Scenario 1:

Let's pretend that you, for whatever reason, maybe a suspected symptom or just to be prudent, head off to your doctor to get a physical check-up or better yet, because of your fear of a heart attack, to see if you have Heart Disease and what is your actual risk of suffering a heart attack.

Your doctor decides to do blood work to find out what your actual serum levels are; good HDL, bad LDL cholesterol and triglycerides. After getting your results back it is apparent that you have too much of the bad stuff such as Low-Density cholesterol and not enough of the good stuff such as High-Density cholesterol, at least according to the 'targeted' published guidelines. He puts you on LDL cholesterol reducing drugs and counsels you on your diet; again in an effort to get you to those published LDL, HDL and triglyceride targets.

If you are really persistent in your quest for more specific answers on your actual risk he may go ahead and give you a stress-test; just 'to be sure'. You pass that baby with flying colors; no chest discomfort at all! You leave feeling awesome with the confidence that only comes from being in the able hands of an expert; in this case your trusted doctor.

All is well, right? Actually, this old guy says NO! All is definitely not right. I will explain in much more clinical and common-sensical detail as you get further into this book.

Scenario 2:

You are enjoying dinner with your family when you are overcome with abdominal pain. You fall to the floor and begin a most nauseating and embarrassing episode of voiding yourself of everything in your stomach and bowels. 911 is called and they transport you to the hospital where they quickly diagnose you with urolithiasis; in your case, Kidney Stones. They give you some sedation while you wait.

The hospital staff summon a Urologist who is an expert at treating the disease and after a short conference he decides to 'stent' you to 'stabilize' you and, more importantly, to prevent the offending kidney stone from moving and causing even more damage and discomfort. He then schedules you for ESWL or Extracorporeal Shock Wave Lithotripsy treatment. He explains the basics of clinical and technical sides of ESWL and further explains the procedure and some of the associated risks; general anesthesia, some possible temporary loss of bladder control as well as residual pain. You should be up and at it in a week or so and back to normal in mere weeks of treatment.

Whether the doctor submits you to the older high-pressure unit or a newer optimized-pressure unit there are many concerns that you should have regarding what is being done for (to?) you, and why.

Again, I will explain in much greater detail in a subsequent chapter on the functionality of the Kidneys and Kidney Disease.

CHAPTER TWO
COMMON SENSE CARDIOLOGY?

"Common sense comes not from education but far too often in spite of education."

They, whoever *they* are, say that you should always start with a bang while others, whoever *others* are, say that you should always close with a bang. I will accommodate both of them, whoever *them* are, and start and finish with a bang.

Before I go any further I want to make sure that there will be no misunderstanding as to where I go with this chapter. I have a lot of respect for most family practitioners and cardiologists. I have the utmost respect for those family practice docs and cardiologists who have placed the patient's well being at the forefront and have adapted Cardiovascular CT in their quest to do what is right and what will provide optimized clinical outcomes for their patients.

Now let's forge ahead. Here is the naked truth about cholesterol and its importance as an indicator of CAD, coronary artery disease; some may even suggest that high LDL cholesterol is actual proof of the disease. Knowledge and Common Sense dictate that this is closer to Hogwash than legitimate.

What if I were to tell you that there are numerous studies out there that pretty well debunk most of the cholesterol hype being bandied around; hype that was carefully word-crafted to do one thing and one thing only; scare the hell out of you and send you running to your family practitioner or cardiologist to get tested for cholesterol levels. The end result is blood work (with its inherent profits) then another follow-up office visit (with its inherent profit) to review your serum levels.

The doctor will sit you down then pick up the file containing your serum results. He will study the results for a while then gaze at you with a most serious look.

"Heart attacks are the number one killer of all people today and you appear to be well on your way to having one. Before we go over these results let me educate you a bit on what we can do to try and avert this potential disaster. The National Cholesterol Education Program sets desired 'target' levels of cholesterol, both the bad low-density type and the good high-density type. They also set 'targets' for triglycerides; these numbers are important and we must work hard to get you to these 'target' levels. You must get down to those levels."

You are now at a point where a prescription will probably be given to you for cholesterol-lowering medication. You leave feeling better thinking that you are headed to a long and healthy life as a result. The doctor and the pharmaceutical company shareholders are also elated because they all made money from their rather questionable marketing program.

Cholesterol levels are definitely a significant factor for something but for screening for CAD; I don't think so.

Medical Facts

> Cholesterol is a waxy, fat-like substance that occurs naturally in all parts of the body and is made by the liver. Cholesterol also is present in foods we eat. People need cholesterol for the body to function normally. Cholesterol is present in the cell walls or membranes everywhere in the body, including the brain, nerves, muscles, skin, liver, intestines, and heart.
>
> HDL (high density lipoprotein) cholesterol is known as good cholesterol. HDL takes the bad cholesterol out of your blood and keeps it from building up in your arteries.
>
> LDL (low density lipoprotein) cholesterol is known as bad cholesterol because it can build up on the walls of your arteries and increase your chances of getting cardiovascular disease. When being tested for high

cholesterol, you want a high HDL number and a low LDL number.

Triglycerides are a type of fat that is found in the blood. They are the most common type of fat and are a major source of energy. When a person eats, his or her body uses the calories it needs for quick energy. It converts excess calories into triglycerides and stores them in fat cells to use later. In normal amounts, triglycerides are very important to good health.

To properly set the stage for the following ponderings let's first take a look at the body's most precious organ; the heart.

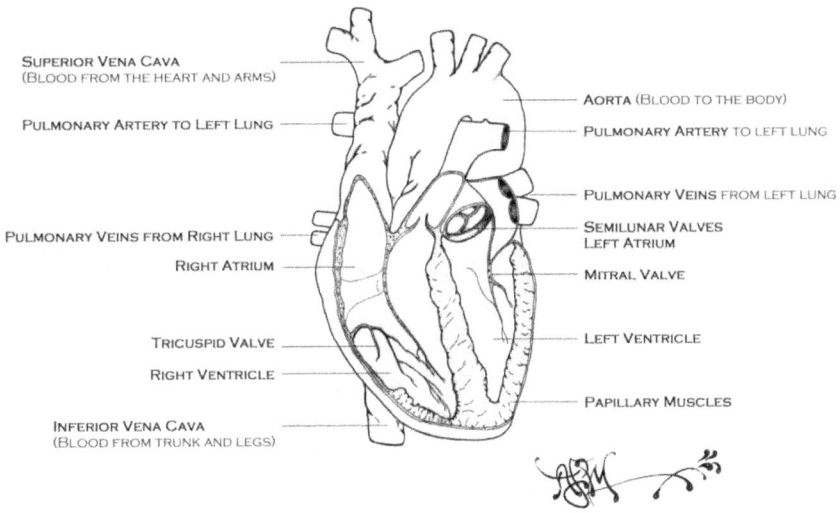

The heart and its function is covered in much greater retail in Chapter Seven of this book.

The heart pumps oxygenated blood to and from the entire body including the heart itself and, of course, the muscles within the heart. This blood is delivered to the muscle of the heart through a series of arteries embedded on the surface of the muscle called coronary arteries.

The greatest threat to the heart and the life that it supports is a heart attack.

Let's explore deeper into the heart and look at exactly what causes heart attacks. Most people think that a heart attack is always accompanied by severe pain and chest discomfort; that is not the case. There are basically two very distinct, but just as threatening, types of heart attacks. In the simplest of terms they are the symptomatic heart attack, that being accompanied by severe pain and an assortment of other negative physical manifestations, and the non-Q-wave or silent non-symptomatic heart attack.

The symptomatic heart attack, or myocardial infarction, is the result of ischemic heart disease. Ischemia occurs when the blood supply to the actual myocardium, the heart muscle itself, is reduced to a point where the myocardium does not receive sufficient oxygen to remain functional.

Contrary to popular belief most myocardial infarctions, commonly referred to as heart attacks, are the result of a non flow-limiting lesion in the artery erupting and releasing a blood clot that lodges downstream where it then stops the flow of blood in the artery of the heart. Blockage of a coronary artery deprives the myocardium of blood and oxygen. If blood is not fully restored within 30 to 40 minutes, the heart muscle will die, resulting in acute heart failure or death.

Symptoms of an MI can include chest pain or discomfort in the center of your chest that comes and goes for minutes at a time, pain or discomfort in the upper body, including the arms, left shoulder, back, neck, jaw or stomach, difficulty breathing or shortness of breath, sweating, a feeling of fullness, indigestion or choking, nausea or vomiting, light headedness or dizziness, extreme weakness or anxiety and rapid or irregular heartbeats.

Most symptomatic MIs produce what is called a 'Q' wave on an ECG.

A precursor to a symptomatic, fatal MI is a silent or non-Q-wave heart attack. A silent heart attack is just that... silent! There is no pain, no dizziness or any other symptoms. The victim is normally totally unaware that anything has happened. The fact that there are no associated symptoms should not be taken lightly. Most people that suffer fatal MIs have had multiple silent, non-Q wave heart attacks prior to the big one.

Medical Tip:

> *Get tested for non-Q wave, so-called 'silent' heart attacks. The healing process of these silent heart attacks leaves scar tissue and calcium deposits that can be easily detected with the proper cardiovascular imaging technology, CVCT.*

Again, contrary to popular belief, Coronary Artery Disease (CAD) is a disease of the vessel wall, not the lumen, or lining, of the vessel. Silent heart attacks occur when soft plaques begin to grow like little pimples embedded just under the inner lining of the blood vessel walls. But instead of pus, these soft plaques are filled with cholesterol and other fats. These plaques are often referred to as "ticking time bombs," because when they rupture they cause injury to the vessel wall. After the rupture, the healing process begins when a blood clot forms at the site of the injury (just as it would if you cut your hand). If the blood clot is large enough, it can suddenly and completely block blood flow to the heart muscle, causing a heart attack that can also lead to sudden death.

Most of the general population has not been educated on the atherosclerotic process and these 'plaque explosions' and thus still do not realize that the majority of these eruptions do not cause chest pains or any other obvious symptoms hence no myocardial infarction. What really happens is that the injury from the rupture simply heals over without notice as the body dispatches healing substances including calcium that form a protective scar that over time becomes calcified. The body, as it does with most injuries, heals itself by trying to create stabilizing bone at the site of the injury.

This calcification is the real key to heart attack prevention for the only natural way that the calcification can be in the coronary artery is through this injury site reparation process.

We have just taken our first step in our common sense approach to dealing with Coronary Artery Disease or Atherosclerosis. Silent heart attacks are far more prevalent than first thought and also far more dangerous than first thought. For any realistic assessment of your risk for a future MI it is absolutely imperative that you determine whether or not you have suffered any 'silent' heart attacks. Ask, no demand that your doctor order a coronary artery calcification (CAC) CT study for you.

Now we can get back to that study regarding cholesterol. In the Sachdeva Study the researchers looked at the admission lipid levels of 136,905 patients from some 500 hospitals. These patients had all been admitted for CAD, myocardial infarctions or heart attacks.

The results were staggering in that 77% of those patients that had cardiac episodes had normal LDL, the bad low-density lipoproteins! 77% were below 130mg/dl!!!

The target for HDL, the good high-density lipoproteins, is 40mg/dl or higher. This study showed that a staggering 45% of these patients had HDL levels of 45mg/dl or higher!

Triglycerides levels showed that nearly half of these victims had triglyceride levels that were well within the target range of 150mg/dl.

The authors of this study concluded that there needs to be further studies to further help determine what levels should be set as targets.

My common sense and skepticism allow me to comfortably offer up a much better answer. This study comprised of a huge number of patients, 136,905, from 541 hospitals over a long term, from 2000 to 2006. It does not take a mental giant, when looking at this huge study from a huge number of hospitals around the globe, to come to one simple and accurate conclusion; statistically the LDL, HDL and triglyceride levels that puts you **most at risk for having**

a cardiac event are the so-called normal level; the very level that the doctors motivate you so fervently to strive for!

I think that you can see why I may be somewhat suspicious of the motives of many who have taken the Hippocratic Oath.

"My good friend and colleague Dr. John Rumberger is somewhat famous for saying "in order to effectively treat heart disease you must first find (manifest) heart disease!" Really, is it not plain old common sense that before anything else regarding any course of therapy for CAD that you first see if the patient *actually has* the disease.

Common Sense Medical Tip:

> *My father, God rest his soul, used to always tell me that you will only be allowed so many 'holes' in your body in a lifetime. Whether these 'holes' result from a gunshot or a planned puncture from a skilled and well-intentioned medical care giver, any one perforation of the skin may well be the one that is the very cause of your demise. The problem is that you never know which one it will be. Common sense dictates that you avoid any and all 'invasive' procedures whenever possible where there is a less-risk-laden, equally effective, non-invasive alternative.*

Let me ask a simple question; who of the following had the greatest risk factors for a heart attack? Sir Winston Churchill who was severely overweight, was a physically wreck and ate and drank to excess far too often; or Jim Fixx, the marathon runner who was extremely fit, the perfect weight and was a non-drinker and non-smoker.

It was sort of a trick question. Jim Fixx died of a heart attack at the age of 53 and Sir Winston lived to the ripe old age of 91. I point this out so that you realize that in today's world it is a gross understatement to say that there is a severe misunderstanding of just how to assess a patient's individual risk for CAD.

That being said, however, there is a very clear answer to this dilemma and John Rumberger had it right.

Below is a diagram of the multitude of risk factors and arterial structure and function tests that are out there to assess your potential for having manifest CAD.

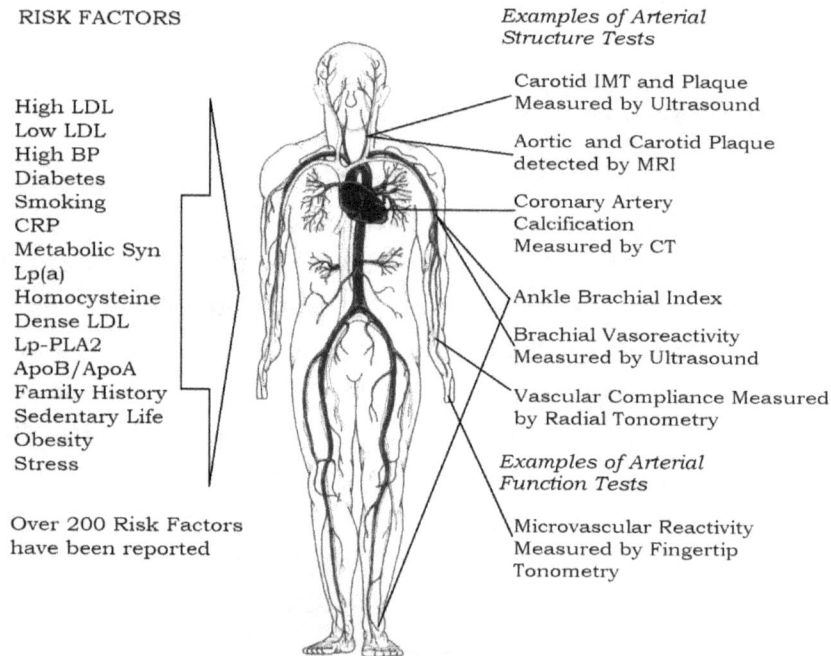

RISK FACTORS

High LDL
Low LDL
High BP
Diabetes
Smoking
CRP
Metabolic Syn
Lp(a)
Homocysteine
Dense LDL
Lp-PLA2
ApoB/ApoA
Family History
Sedentary Life
Obesity
Stress

Over 200 Risk Factors have been reported

Examples of Arterial Structure Tests

Carotid IMT and Plaque Measured by Ultrasound

Aortic and Carotid Plaque detected by MRI

Coronary Artery Calcification Measured by CT

Ankle Brachial Index

Brachial Vasoreactivity Measured by Ultrasound

Vascular Compliance Measured by Radial Tonometry

Examples of Arterial Function Tests

Microvascular Reactivity Measured by Fingertip Tonometry

One of these tests, the Coronary Artery Calcification study by CT, is a well-known, inexpensive, readily available, non-invasive, single breath-hold study that actually detects, identifies and quantifies definite (manifest) CAD within a patient. The study can be completed in about five minutes. The sole etiology of Coronary Artery Calcification (CAC) is CAD; the presence of CAC means that you have the disease, plain and simple. Conversely, the lack of CAC in a patient puts that patient at absolute minimal risk of having the disease.

This CAC study is one of the biggest no-brainers that this old guy has ever seen! When I had the two CV Imaging/CAC study centers in Florida we saw tons (literally) of patients with grossly elevated cholesterol levels that had clean arteries and no CAD as well as many, many with so-called normal cholesterol that had significant CAD! As I stated cholesterol may be looked at as a risk factor for the disease but if you want to know for sure if you have this killer disease get scanned for CAC; just use your own God given common sense!

"A parade is really only a parade if there is a leader and some followers."

The routine disregard by the medical community for this study is truly outrageous and the stated reasons are also outrageous. Here we are talking about CAD, the number one killer of mankind and the ability to reign in its devastation. The main reason for disregarding CAC scanning that they use is that there is residual radiation after the test. The radiation levels of this study are far less than the 'background' radiation one would get from living in Miami for a year. Common sense risk/reward evaluation is where my brain goes: do I want to absorb a miniscule amount of additional radiation to find the disease early or take the chance of actually dying from the disease? Give me a break.... like I said it is a no-brainer!

That brings up the question of exactly why the medical community at large really seems to look the other way when it comes to this life-saving study? I hate to be the bearer of bad news here but you simply have to "follow the bouncing dollars" as another of my colleagues, Carter Newton says. Remember my caveat of replacing 'doctor's practice' with 'business' and 'patient' with 'client'. The doctors make far more money going on their more routine, 'gold-standard', far less-effective 'risk factor' fishing expeditions.

The question of what to do after you have confirmed Coronary Artery Disease is a most difficult one.

There are a host of therapeutic options ranging from simple medication, diet and life-style changes to surgical and mechanical intervention.

There is another option that is readily available yet widely ignored by the traditional medical community. Chelation therapy is in many cases a viable alternative; one which unfortunately is not a very popular one with cardiologists. The vast majority of the cardiology community view chelation as nothing more than 'Voodoo' quackery. They refuse to even consider its potential. They do so, however, recognizing that they all have in reality prescribed chelation medication to their patients; they do so routinely in the form of oral chelation of acetylsalicylic acid, Aspirin.

Voodoo medicine or non-Voodoo medicine? I guess it depends on just who is dispensing the medicine!

CHAPTER THREE
VOODOO MEDICINE

"What cannot easily be explained with traditional wisdom is most often even more easily cast aside as pure idiocy!"

More than 60% of all health care dollars spent in this country last year were doled out for alternative medicine; chiropractic, holistic, homeopathic, acupuncture, chelation, etc.

The majority of the population are increasingly turning to alternative medicine because it allows them a better opportunity to personally manage their health care, it's cheaper and most importantly, in the majority of cases it provides a much more satisfactory outcome; in other words it works!

Most in the mainstream health care delivery system look at alternative medicine as nothing more than unprofessional, laughable, snake-oil-salesman-type quackery; Voodoo medicine. Voodoo medicine which to them, unfortunately, is competing rather successfully for their patients' dollars.

I must admit that I was amongst the naysayers in days gone by. Whenever I hear the term Voodoo I recall years ago when I was on a business trip with my wife, God bless her soul (no, she is not dead but is still voluntarily living with me, poor thing!) to the 'Big Easy', New Orleans, Louisiana. We were wandering down Bourbon Street with Jacques Lafitte's bar as the semi-ultimate destination; the Bourbon Orleans hotel hopefully being the final spot for the night. About a block away from the bar is the famous Marie Laveau's Voodoo shop. My wife, knowing full well what my feelings regarding Voodoo were at the time, insisted that we go in and explore the darker side of Bourbon Street; if it is possible for that particular street to have anything less than a darker side. I, somewhat hesitantly, went up the stairs with her and into the smoke-filled establishment. Much to our amazement, we ended up face to face with the mistress of the occult herself, Marie Laveau. My lovely wife Marsha quickly got into a 'dark' conversation with

Laveau regarding some Poltergeists that used to inhabit my lovely, but often somewhat strange wife's, old house. It did not take long for the 'Lady in Black' to determine that I was nothing, if I were not a total non-believer in this Voodoo stuff. She immediately threw a Voodoo 'pox' on me and asked me to leave. I started to laugh but she responded in a very Poltergeist sounding, sort of possessed Linda Blair voice; "you will be a believer, and it will be very, very soon indeed."

I really couldn't take anymore anyway so to keep the peace I headed to the door, turned around and told Marsha that I would be waiting for her outside. I then turned toward the stairs and took a step. It was like somebody had tied my ankles together; I went head over heels down the stairs and landed with an unceremonious thud on my back on the sidewalk in front of all who roamed Bourbon Street to see. I remember looking up and hearing that demonic voice once again laughing, emanating from up those damned stairs deep inside the bowels of that dark, smoky building while I gathered my thoughts on the concrete. Had I just experienced a lesson in the realities of supernatural Voodoo at the hands of Marie Laveau or was it the 6 Hurricanes that I had consumed earlier at Pat O'Brien's that caused my impromptu and faulty Fred Astaire impersonation? I'll never know for sure but I do know that my eyes were forced open a little more to the possibilities of the occult being real after that!

My 'clinical' eyes were forced completely open to the unbelievable results of Voodoo medicine later in life when I had the cardiovascular imaging centers in Florida in the late 90s. My Voodoo medicine 'blinders' actually started getting pulled back much earlier in the 80s by a wonderful master of chiropractic medicine in Orlando. I was invited into the world of alternative medicine by Dr. Dan after fate placed us next to each other on a crowded flight from Boston to Orlando. The flight took more than a couple of hours which allowed us ample time to share thoughts and ideas and plant the seeds on how we could further advance our roles in the health care delivery system if we were to team up.

Dr. Dan turned out to be an absolute gift to all who fell, no pun intended, under his care or those who were guided through their medical careers by his teachings; me being one of the latter. I have always considered it an honor to have been taught so much by this man.

Dr. Dan was a true master of all things neuro-musculal-skeletal. He was one of the very first adapters of a marvelous technology for the alleviation of back pain; the VaxD technology. I often referred to this technology as a modern day 'Rack' because it required the ankles to be secured and the upper torso to be 'stretched' by a computer controlled device. This was the only technology that had been validated and approved by the FDA; the unit would pull the spinal column back into position actually generating a negative pressure in the process which would subsequently pull the injured disk back into place. The end result was a pain-free back patient. Dan was a perfect fit in my 'mission' because he provided superior patient outcomes through the programmed utilization of superior technologies; VaxD being among them.

His systematic approach would result, in relatively short periods of time, freeing people from their debilitating back, neck, shoulder, any structural related problems. People who had been stricken with pain for years would over time be freed from their canes, crutches and, occasionally, even wheelchairs; like I said Dr. Dan was one awesome guy! As adjunct services he also offered acupuncture and nutritional therapies. He was, above all, a DC, Doctor of Chiropractic. A quack, a charlatan, a Voodoo medicine man; I think NOT!

It was Dan who introduced me to the ERE method of clinical practice. *Evaluate* the patient to make sure that you fully understand, and are treating, the real problem; *Rehabilitate* to bring the patient back to as close to normal as possible; then *Educate* the patient to avoid re-injury. This is such a logical process for physicians to follow because it is an exercise in common sense! You would be amazed at the number of doctors out there who do not follow anything resembling these simple guiding clinical principles.

> *"The doctor of the future will give no medicine but instead will interest his patients in the care of the human frame, in diet, and in the cause and prevention of disease."*
> — THOMAS EDISON

Dr. Dan was also a very staunch proponent of yet another of the so-called 'fringe' medical practices; chelation therapy.

> *Chelation (pronounced key-LAY-shun) is the use of a chemical substance to bind molecules, such as metals or minerals, and hold them tightly so they can be removed from the body. Chelation has been scientifically proven to remove excess or toxic metals before they can cause damage to the body. It was first used in the 1940's by the Navy to treat lead poisoning.*
>
> *The most common form of chelation therapy uses a man-made amino acid called EDTA (ethylene diamine tetra acetic acid). EDTA removes heavy metals and minerals from the blood, such as lead, iron, copper, and calcium, and is approved by the FDA for treating lead poisoning and poisoning from other heavy metals.*
>
> *During the normal chelation treatment, a needle is inserted into the patient's vein, which is connected to an intravenous (IV) drip containing EDTA. A typical session is about 3 hours long, and they are scheduled 1 to 3 times a week. Twenty to 30 sessions are usually necessary. Oral, non-IV based chelation also exists.*

Although I had seen some pretty impressive results when I was with Dr. Dan in the late 80s, the real miraculous results of chelation therapy would only become apparent to me in our cardiovascular imaging center in the late 90s.

Our CVCT center in Sarasota specialized in Coronary Artery Scanning for the detection, identification and quantification of CAD by detecting calcium in the arteries. We could find early, manifest or pre-symptomatic CAD at a point where it could be arrested or even reversed; normally through medication and/or lifestyle changes.

> *Coronary Artery Calcification (CAC) is the direct result of small, non-stenotic lesions erupting during silent heart attacks. The body's healing process creates calcium (bone). The sole etiology of CAC is CAD! If you have calcium in the arteries, you have CAD, or Atherosclerosis! The higher the calcium levels the greater the risk to the patient of a potentially fatal Q-wave or symptomatic heart attack.*

Whenever we found atherosclerosis in a patient we would have an obligatory discussion with them confirming our findings. It was inevitable that the question of what they could do about the disease would come up. Depending on the CAC quantification levels of the patient there was a wide range of options. As the calcification quantification levels rose, however, the list of reasonable options unfortunately diminished. One of the choices that remained for those higher-risk patients was chelation.

In the planning stages for the center I had met a doctor in Sarasota, a PHD, who specialized in oral nutritional chelation. I immediately contracted with him to provide his expertise to the patients of our center. We developed a program whereby he would run some serum studies on the higher-risk patient then, based upon their personal calcium score, age, weight, etc. would create a personalized nutritional chelating cocktail to be ingested in prescribed amounts over a specific time frame.

The calcium levels in a patient determined their risk for a future event. A score of 100 or less normally carried the lowest risk with a score of 200 to 300 being high and anything over 400 requiring immediate medical attention.

We had one particular patient, a male in his mid-fifties who was a local executive in the health care industry. As a professional courtesy we had extended an invitation to him to get scanned for CAC; he, most fortunately, accepted our offer.

He appeared to be in pretty fair physical shape, good medical history, exercised regularly, was a mild drinker and did not smoke. We expected to find some calcium, maybe in the 200-300 range but what we found blew us all away. This healthy looking, great feeling guy had a CAC score over 1300, the second or third highest that I had ever heard of! We immediately called two people; firstly, our Medical Director, a cardiologist, and; the second person was David, our nutritional/chelation specialist.

Unfortunately there were few reasonable surgical options. After many, many hours of reviewing the scans we, along with the patient and Dr. David, decided on a course of immediate action. David went to work and within a day or so had a personalized concoction for our patient. Because of the hyper-high levels of CAC there was an absolute immediate need to do something. It was also imperative that we determine the efficacy of the treatment in as timely a manner as possible. The patient agreed to a plan where we would circumvent our normal operational restrictions on serial scanning. We would rescan him in 4-6 months; just to be sure that we were actually positively affecting his condition.

At the end of the fifth month we rescanned the patient and again, we were blown away; his score had dropped from 1300 to just over 900. After another scan a year later he was at just over 600!

Was Dr. David a quack, a charlatan, a snake-oil-salesman practicing Voodoo medicine? You be the judge; for me I say hell no! There is no question in my mind that chelation therapy definitely works.

David had another patient that had contacted him when we had the centers. He was an older gentleman who had diabetes and had been battling an infection of his lower right leg and foot. I had the great fortune to be there when the man arrived at David's office. What prompted the call was that his traditional doctor had 'thrown in the towel' and wanted to schedule the man for immediate amputation. David was to be his last resort and David, thank God, took him on.

About three months later I was out for dinner at a fine restaurant where there was a nice band and a dance floor; there he was, the old guy, dancing his heart out with both of his natural legs and feet!

Again, chelation works; maybe not always, but in the right hands when it does it renders miraculous results.

Common Sense Medical Tip:

> EDTA (ethylene diamine tetra-acetic acid) is the common agent used in chelation therapy for a host of reasons; it rids the arterial system of heavy metals and calcium. It is also contains properties that protect the lining of the arteries.
>
> The closest thing to EDTA that is readily available to you is regular white vinegar; it has a chemical structure that is close to the structure of both EDTA and acetylsalicylic acid (ASA) or common aspirin.
>
> The Mediterranean Diet is definitely healthy for you but why; because of the veggies? Partly, but I propose that the major benefit is from the salad dressing, mainly the vinegar. Pickles are pickles because they are in vinegar. Vinegar, like EDTA and Aspirin, is good for you and your arterial system; eat a lot of pickles; hell, go ahead and drink the pickle juice while you are at it.
>
> "A pickle a day may very well keep the doctor at bay." Try it; who doesn't like pickles!

CHAPTER FOUR
TRADITIONAL (NON-VOODOO?) MEDICINE

"Common sense is a very elusive beast indeed escaping from far too many of the very brightest minds of our leaders."

I reiterate that the world owes a huge debt of gratitude to those medical specialists that were the early adapters of Cardiovascular CT for early detection of CAD as well as for non-invasive CT Angiography in their personal quest to do what is right for their patients. Doctors such as Jim Adams, Carter Newton, Paolo Raggi, John Rumberger, Chris Becker, Alan Guerci, Warren Janowitz, Art Agatston, Yadon Arad; the list goes on and on. Without these CVCT pioneers there would be little light at the end of the cardiovascular disease tunnel. Today, thanks to them the light shines brightly and the numbers of adapters continues to grow and hopefully society may very well see the actual eradication of this devastating disease.

Forging ahead in the sometimes ugly area of clinical realty; remember the litany of fine, flowering comments about me at the very beginning of this book; words which formed the very cornerstone upon which I built my case for your respect and trust. Well, sadly, I suspect that after this chapter is read and digested that the accolades may dwindle somewhat. They will drop off precipitously not as a result of the content not being totally accurate but as the result of me taking my literary clinical 'sword' out of its sheath and tastefully using it to 'gore the oxen' as they say of the majority of cardiologists out there. So be it.

Who is committing the greatest offense; a quack, charlatan, snake-oil-salesman rendering what could very well be good medicine or a preeminent medical specialist consciously doling out what he knows to be inferior medicine? It's a trick question that sets the stage for this chapter.

Remember Carter Newton's caveat about following the 'bouncing dollar' when it comes to health care strategies and clinical behavior that common sense and knowledge dictates that it runs against the Hippocratic Oath and the supposed intended goal of the provision of superior patient outcomes.

Medical Facts:
The Hippocratic Oath is an oath historically taken by physicians. It is one of the most widely known of Greek medical texts. In its original form, it requires a new physician to swear, by a number of healing gods, to uphold specific ethical standards.

Let's again visit the number one killer of men and women in the Western World; cardiovascular disease, especially Myocardial Infarctions, or MIs.

CVD Statistics:
CAD kills 500,000 Americans annually!

The mean biological onset of CAD in the US is now *11 years of age*!

Heart Disease kills more women annually than the next 7 causes of death <u>combined</u>!

There are 875,000 *symptomatic* myocardial infarctions annually

For 50% of Americans the *first and only* symptom of CAD is a myocardial infarction!

Approximately 50% of 1st MI victims die.

Most fatal MIs are the result of a *non flow-limiting lesion* erupting.

There are estimated to be in excess of 200,000 <u>silent</u>, non Q-wave heart attacks annually!

These non Q-wave attacks normally leave residual small extra-lumenal calcific lesions.

The majority of non Q-wave heart attack victims have no idea that they have suffered damage and have a 17-fold risk of death from heart disease than those without heart damage.

The most important statistic is the fact that over half of all who die from a heart attack do so with the very first and only symptom being death! Most never even know they had the disease! We must, as a global community, not only find better ways of assessing risk for MI, but also integrate and utilize these superior technologies in a *real* fight against this disease.

We've already looked at the so-called 'gold standards' for risk factor assessment and arterial structure and function tests so now let's look at the so-called 'gold standards' for high-risk, or suspected high-risk, non-symptomatic and symptomatic patients. Keep in mind that even though you feel fine, unless you see a physician, *a physician who utilizes the proper technologies*, you will never know for sure.

Here is an illustration of the different methods for assessment and their diagnostic sensitivity;

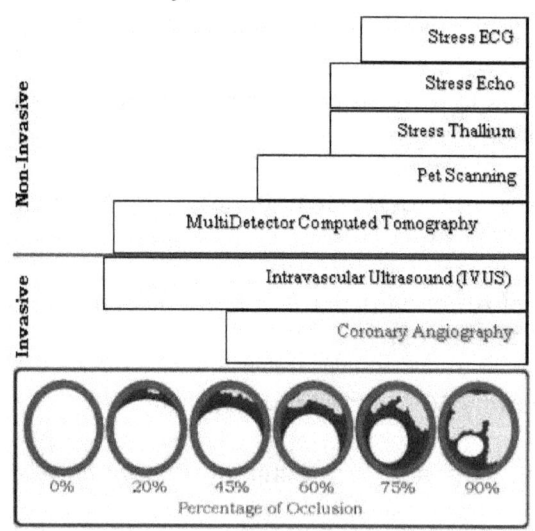

I routinely used this chart in my lectures. It shows a cross section of an artery with the degree of CAD involvement and the ability of the different technologies to detect CAD at that level.

The most often used tests for heart disease detection are stress tests and direct coronary angiography; stress testing is non-invasive and the real 'gold standard', angiography is very invasive carrying its own involved risks.

This chart clearly illustrates the problem in today's cardiovascular detection world. Present day 'gold standards' for the effective detection and assessment of CVD are grossly inadequate as they are heavily dependent upon hemodynamic changes in the coronary arteries; a change that only starts to be detectable during the latter, less risky stages of the disease.

Common sense and clinical knowledge tells us that in order to effectively treat CVD you must first find the disease; and the earlier the better.

Another of the key statistics is the fact that most fatal MIs are the result of a non-flow limiting lesion erupting. A non-flow limiting lesion is normally one which is less than a 50% occlusive and would never be detectable utilizing the so-called 'gold standards'!

Medical Fact:
The heart is a self-architecting organ! The heart will over sufficient time develop collateral blood flow to make up for diminishing blood flow to its muscle. The heart will also change the structure of its arteries to compensate for the initial invasion of extra-lumenal lesions into the lumen, or inner lining of the vessel; this is called 'remodeling'.

Coronary artery disease is a disease of the vessel wall. Lesions that form are extra-lumenal and as a direct result of vessel remodeling the lumen, remains relatively unaffected which renders the lesion undetectable by today's so-called 'gold standards'!

> Direct angiography and stress testing will not detect the normal non-blood flow limiting, extra-lumenal, 'culprit' lesion; the exact lesion type that is responsible for the vast majority of fatal MIs!!

If I know this believe me just about every cardiologist, cardiology radiologist and cardiovascular specialist on the globe does also! I ain't no Einstein and, if they really don't know this, they most certainly should and probably should not be practicing medicine.

This brings up what is probably the most significant question of this whole exercise. Why would a well educated cardiologist, fully recognizing the all-too-obvious deficiencies of the present so-called 'gold standards' for CVD detection and assessment, continue to risk his/her patient's well being by utilizing inferior, ineffective technologies and methodologies when he/she is fully aware of, and has unfettered access to superior, far more effective technologies and associated methodologies?

In the case of stress testing and angiography there is an even greater clinical and ethical dilemma. These tests only get 'triggered' by significant stenoses (>50%) and cannot detect the more lethal smaller 'culprit' lesions. As a result of these major deficiencies a negative study in no way converts to clean arteries or non-threatening CAD; it only means that whatever lesions exist have not yet progressed to a point where they impede the flow of blood.

That's why we so often hear of people dropping dead of a heart attack within hours or days of having been given a 'clean bill of health' as a result of undergoing a negative stress test or angiographic exam! We all should remember Tim Russert, the newscaster who a few years back was provided with the so-called 'gold standard' of care; a recently performed 'clean' stress test; Statin medication; Aspirin, Ace Inhibitors and, even more important if you recall previous chapters, reached his doctor recommended 'target' lipid profiles. Tim died within mere days of undergoing and passing a stress test; he died of a massive heart attack! Tim was 58 when he passed.

Medical Fact:
More than half of those who present at an Emergency Department with chest pain are in fact not suffering from a heart attack or any cardiac related event instead anguish from esophageal reflux or some other non-life threatening event.

My wife recently woke me up and said that she had some chest discomfort. After giving her a couple of aspirins I quickly loaded her into the car and rushed off to our local hospital's Emergency Department. After the normal blood-letting and ECG/telemetry hook up we sat there waiting. The ECG was not showing any signs of cardiac stress and her arterial blood gas levels were good as were her color and all other vital signs.

Within an hour or so the ER doctor came in and said that all looked great but, just to be sure, Marsha should undergo an immediate stress test. I asked why? The doctor looked at me with that 'how dare you question me' stare. Again I asked why, what would a stress test possibly reveal that would assist her at that moment in making a decision regarding Marsha's immediate risk?

This doctor had no answer that made any clinical sense really seeming unaware that stress testing is designed specifically to identify those at longer-term risk with advanced ischemia, not short-term risk from manifest CAD, follow the money!

There is a great article in Emergency Physicians Monthly on this exact issue by Dr. David Newman of Columbia University.

Before Marsha was discharged I had the opportunity to again engage the doctor and discuss the use of CAC scanning in the ED specifically to rule out the heart as the culprit. A clean CAC study means that there is a less than 1% chance of that patient having a cardiac event within the short-term and they can be discharged with absolute clinical confidence. She had not a clue about CAC!

It really is scary! Just use your common sense; this is not rocket science. Just follow Carter's 'bouncing' dollar bill and replace the word *cardiologist* with 'business owner' and *patient* with 'client'! I have been doing battle with those who routinely perform these somewhat unethical and quasi-illegal procedures for years and years now. Arterial stenting, by-pass grafting and all of their other risk-laden procedures that may, or may not, alleviate symptoms for a while and are totally unnecessary in a tremendous percentage of cases. What we definitely do know, however, is that just about all of these patients will require additional invasive interventions down the line as a direct result of the unavoidable luminal damage and subsequent re-stenosis caused by the very procedures performed by the same cardiologists who have taken the Hippocratic Oath. They are supposed to be doing nothing less than arresting or reversing the disease; not adding to it!

"Regrettably even the greatest of cardiovascular specialists are not immune to heart attacks nor, even more regrettably, are they immune to 'ethical challenge'!"

A.J. Mueller

CHAPTER FIVE
MAY THE (MAGNETIC) FORCE BE WITH YOU!

"Common sense is like physical beauty; most who are lacking in them have not a clue of same."

Providence is awesome... sometimes. It was 1983 and I, through a rather strange series of planned and spontaneous events and occurrences, found myself in a corporate meeting in New Jersey between several executives and clinical specialists from a number of hospitals in the United States and some top American executives from Siemens Medical out of Germany. Siemens had developed a new imaging technology that had been recently been cleared by the Food and Drug Administration (FDA) for routine clinical imaging applications on humans in the USA. The technology was truly awesome; borderline miraculous. It allowed for non-invasive imaging of organs and surrounding structures deep within the anatomy with unbelievable resolution and image quality. The only other way to see the target structures with such quality and physical integrity would be to surgically remove the organs which, in reality, would have been somewhat detrimental to the future health of the patient. Additionally, surgical removal would not have been as desirable as a result of the unavoidable damage to the tissue surrounding the surgical site.

The executives from Siemens and the hospitals fully recognized the unbelievable clinical benefits to both the clinicians and their patients; for the very first time clinical and research medical professionals could inspect the inner workings of a human being in a quick, non-invasive, non-radiating study! They were in a quandary, actually totally dumbfounded, however, resulting from the fact that the marketplace was not responding in a very positive way to this new miraculous, medical imaging breakthrough.

How did this awesome technology work? In the simplest of terms the most abundant compound in the human body is hydrogen which has a very simple atomic structure; a positively charged proton and a single negatively charged spinning electron. By applying a magnetic force to the targeted area these electrons align themselves then, by applying different sound waves of varying frequencies, the electrons resonate at different rates allowing the on-board computer's algorithms to pick up these signals and create the rather spectacular images of the targeted organs.

I had done my homework; the personal feedback from the many clinicians who had tested this technology was that, at least in their professional minds, much of the reluctance was patient-driven. To perform a study required that the patient be placed on a sliding table and passed through a relatively small bore in the large gantry. It was problematic for both claustrophobic and non-claustrophobic patients. Claustrophobia aside, they were facing an even bigger challenge in convincing the rather skeptical patients to get on the table and voluntarily go through a machine that had its technical name emblazoned on the gantry.... *Nuclear* Magnetic Resonance was there in full view right over where the patient was going to be passed through; NUCLEAR Magnetic Resonance!

These highly-paid, mental giants of the medical-imaging industry, in their quest to rapidly get the technology to market had not even considered the fear that anything named Nuclear would place in the minds of most American people. After much more reality checking, discussions and suggestions from me and my colleagues they reluctantly caved in and Nuclear Magnetic Resonance became the much more benign sounding Magnetic Resonance Imaging, or as it is more commonly referred to today, MRI.

Once the equipment had been renamed and re-introduced MRI became an absolute must at all medical facilities. The doctors everywhere were writing orders for the study on almost all of their patients; even those who really did not need an MRI study; a somewhat normal but highly undesirable consequence of the introduction of most awesome technologies.

For the sake of honesty, even though we had appeared to be an absolute genius in creative medical marketing, the reality piece was that we had come up with this re-naming solution serendipitously just prior to the time that the American Government was introducing the Diagnostic Related Group or DRG system into the US health care system.

The DRG system forced all hospitals and their privileged physicians, under severe financial penalties, to be far more accurate in the actual diagnosis of the patient upon admission to a hospital. The only realistic method of achieving this was through the forced utilization of superior technologies allowing for clearer non-invasive imaging of the inner organs of the body with the emerging MRI technology. In reality even though I and a few other medical marketing 'experts' took a couple of corporate victory laps the real reason NMR took off after the name change to MRI was the introduction of the national DRG system. As I said, sometimes providence is awesome!

Not only did the men and their magnificent scanning machines not foresee the problematic nature of the name but they grossly underestimated the potential dangers of having such powerful magnetic forces in non laboratory settings, settings such as hospitals, clinics and free-standing and mobile imaging centers.

Once these multi-ton beasts are delivered, installed and turned on the magnet is always on. When the normal person thinks of magnets they usually think of the kind that you played with when young or the magnets that you put on the refrigerator.

To illustrate the actual strength of the magnetic force surrounding an MRI machine as well as a prime example of just how ignorant the manufacturers were regarding their equipment when first introduced I will recount one of my first actual hands-on experiences with a free-standing MRI center.

"Remember that the TITANIC was built by professionals!"

It was in the mid 80's and I was living in Orlando, Florida. My brother and I had been approached by a group of investors who wanted my assistance in putting together a privately owned and operated MRI center in Altamonte Springs, just outside of Orlando proper.

We went through months and months of legal filing of paperwork for permitting and construction. One of the investors had a brand new, very beautiful, very prestigious office building about one-half mile from a major hospital; this would be where they would put the their impressive MRI center. The building was a 'stilted' type with the office space above an open parking garage. Over time we assisted in the negotiation of contracts for service as well as for the equipment. After the space was 'built out' specifically for an imaging center it was time for the installation of the essential equipment. The medical equipment 'riggers' lifted the multi-ton main unit from the truck and placed it carefully through a hole in the upper wall and onto its base where it would rest. It took a few more weeks to reconstruct the wall and to connect all of the electrical cables, computers and all of the support equipment. Finally it was time to 'fire 'er up' and test that beast. The lead technician for Siemens hit the on button and all hell broke loose! The equipment started to shake and vibrate; there were unbelievable clunking sounds emanating from below then, with a tremendous cracking sound, the floor started caving in and fortunately for all of us, the power went off as we all headed for the hills.

The noises coming from below were combinations of the metal floor trusses and bracing bending and cracking as well as a couple of compact cars that had been pulled through the parking lot and lodged up against and entwined with the failed sub-structure.

In retrospect there was absolutely no mystery to what had caused this disaster; the company had never told anyone about the absolute requirement to use only non-ferrous steel in the building; ferrous metals contain iron, a highly magnetic substance. This small omission, combined with the contractors' negligence in not shielding the floor under the scanner allowed this tremendous man-made magnetic force to invade the neighboring environment with somewhat disastrous results.

The imaging center never opened its doors for business and the building had to go through years of redesign and reconstruction to be habitable, however, the Boston Avenue MRI center went down in Imaging Center development infamy; at least no one was killed in this fiasco, unlike many other MRI mishaps.

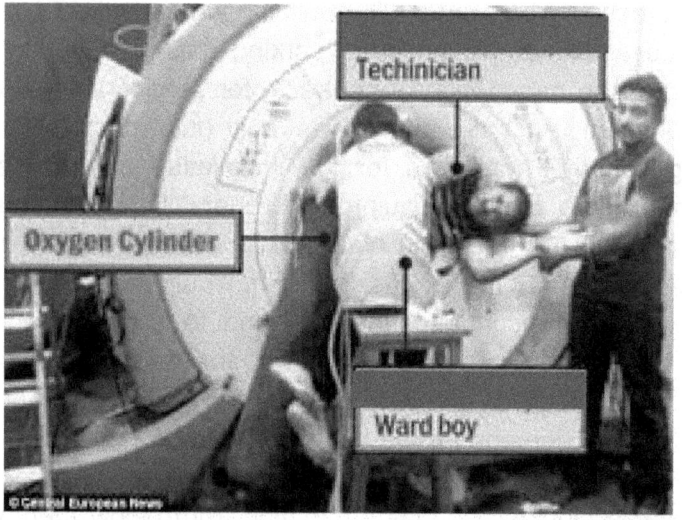

When the very first MRI was installed in a major University Hospital in Los Angeles they soon discovered a couple major issues in the designing and constructing of MRI facilities.

Firstly; make sure that the unit is well RF shielded and as far away as possible from the surgical implant ward and, secondly, make sure that the bore of the machine, where the main magnetic force is created, is not in line with the door to the unit.

When they fired up the machine (I should refrain from any term containing 'fire' for reasons that will soon be obvious!) the resultant magnetic force gathered up everything containing ferrous metal compounds that were not fully secured including pens, paper-clips and heavier items such as chairs and tables turning them all into killer projectiles, and pulled them straight through the door and into the bore of the machine. Those metal objects that were somewhat secured and somewhat distant from the unit, such as pacemakers and other medical implants, were either pulled completely out of their human carriers or displaced, neither of which, as you can imagine, is in the best long-term interest of these unsuspecting victims of 'positive medical ignorance'.

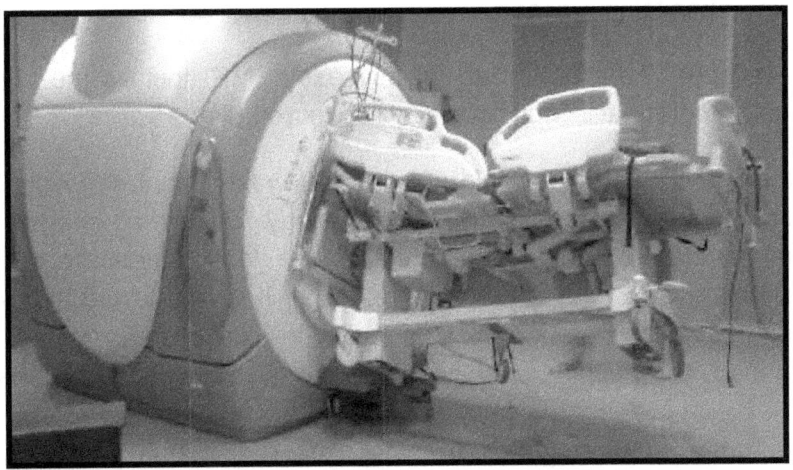

A few years back there was a young boy of six or seven years of age who came to his most unfortunate, untimely demise while undergoing a 'routine' MRI study. For some reason there was a heavy, metal oxygen tank that broke loose from its anchors and was sucked into the bore of the machine like a missile, the exact same spot that the little boy occupied. Although I write about these medical 'miscues' in a humorous manner this is a very, very serious matter indeed.

There was a hospital in the Midwestern US that was installing a new MRI in the brand new 'wing' of the hospital. MRI units are known to make noise and vibrate when in use, and this unit was no different. During testing of the magnet the techs noticed that bolts that were holding the clip for the IV apparatus on the gantry were continually working loose. The answer you ask? 'Let's get the welder who is working down the hall to come in and spot-weld the bolts; they will never work loose then," was the call from the main installation tech. When the welder with his acetylene tank opened the RF shielded door the tank took off like a missile into the bore of the unit. Unfortunately, as it hit the gantry the regulator valve broke off and it not only exploded in flames but the compressed gas within the tank presented a stronger force than the magnetic field and the tank took off like a flaming torpedo turning the multi-million dollar, technologically superior new wing of the hospital into ashes.

Even after years and years of successful MRI installs the high-tech 'gremlins' still occasionally creep in and play.

I recall an event in the mid 90's when I was in final negotiations with Siemens for an emerging technology for cardiac imaging. I was invited to meet with some of the local execs from the company to discuss my pioneering deal. It was decided that we would meet at a brand new MRI facility in Lake Mary, a suburb of Orlando, where they were going to test the newly installed MRI. The facility was magnificent with absolutely no expense spared. It sat a few hundred yards from I-4, the major highway through Central Florida. We had been there a half hour or so when they decided it was time to power up the magnet. After a few minutes of making the common noises MRIs make we could hear terrible crashing sounds from outside the facility that continued for minutes. "That must be one hell of an accident on the highway," said one of the execs. We decided to go out back to see the carnage that supposedly was taking place on I-4. When we went around the building we could see that the crashing was not at all coming from the highway; it was instead being created by every motorcycle, light vehicle and the umpteen dumpsters in the vicinity being yanked into the 'force' and stacked up like toys, a couple of stories high, against the back wall of the facility. Again oversight of essential guidelines had failed and, for whatever reasons, proper shielding had not been installed.

CHAPTER SIX
'FROGGY' LITHO

"Meaningful, useful education often-times comes from the most unusual of places."

Although my strategically planned initial foray into the world of medicine began in the Fall of 1978 my interest in disease and therapeutic remedies actually began many, many years earlier. Back to the mid 1950s my Mother, God rest her soul, was stricken by urolithiasis, a disease of the urinary tract, in her case manifesting itself as totally debilitating kidney-stones. She was taken away and hospitalized where they successfully surgically removed the obstructive stones. After surgery she was bedridden for weeks, went through weeks more of painful recovery and even more months of not being able to function normally.

On many occasions afterwards, when I was still just a young lad, for whatever reason, she would recount the traumatic details of this incapacitating episode to me and, again for whatever reason, it resonated in my brain throughout my more mentally-formative years.

There was another image that, for whatever even stranger reason, had also left an indelible mark on my developing brain. When I was a teenager my Father (I will refrain from using the 'God rest his sole' for a host of reasons one or two of the main ones having been, most unfortunately, discovered by my Mother) had a hunting lodge in the Adirondack Mountains in Northern New York State. Dad was an avid hunter and gun owner and he and I spent a lot of time at the lodge doing a wide variety of things ranging from fishing and hunting to building rock walls and other structures on the property. We used to also spend a lot of time target shooting and talking; with few subjects being off limits.

Dad was a very intelligent guy with a strong knowledge and background in engineering and medicine. Scores of our conversations, fortunately for me, reflected upon many of his own life's experiences; he was also a very, very interesting guy. One particular day we were sitting on the porch overlooking the Salmon River which ran almost straight down the property directly in front of the lodge. There was a normal post-type fence separating the river from the road. Dad had his favorite high-powered rifle on the table. It was a beautiful gun; a 300H&H Magnum with a multi-grained Weatherby stock. He also had a large metal can on the table. He said that he was going to demonstrate some of the laws of physics to me. He did so in a somewhat weird, but comically interesting manner.

"Take this can, fill it with water and put it on top of one of those fence posts down by the street. When you are done go down to the river and get a couple frogs and dump them into the can."

Knowing Dad, I knew that whatever it was that was going to happen next would most likely far surpass being just comically interesting. I was right but it took years and years, actually a quarter of a century of my life and fateful external circumstances for me to fully realize that this one occurrence was the basis for what turned out to be a truly pivotal moment in my life.

Can in hand I went through the yard, across the road, through the gate and down to the river where I filled the container with water then carried it back to the fence, carefully placing it atop one of the posts. I then went back and carefully gathered up two wonderful specimens of local frogs and even more carefully placed them in the can. I hate to admit it but I had a feeling that these little guys' time on earth was about to come to an end so I somewhat secretly said a goodbye to each as I plunked them into the round, water-filled tin retainer. I then quickly walked back up to the porch where my Father sat patiently with an air of total confidence surrounding him.

He then slowly, almost theatrically, loaded the rifle with bullets; big bullets that really resembled small, shiny rockets.

"Son, you are now about to see a lesson in transferring energy from this gun to the water down there in those cans."

He then went on to explain that water is very dense; so dense in fact that, unless frozen, it cannot be condensed. He went on to explain how any force applied to the water, in this case as a result of the impact from the bullet, will generate a shock wave which will then be transferred through the water with minimal loss in strength and affect everything in its path. Sort of made sense to me.

"Our unsuspecting guests, the frogs, are sort of unwilling participants who will share some good fortune and, unfortunately, bad fortune in this demonstration. The good news is that these simple amphibious creatures will be among the luckiest, if not the luckiest, of all of the non-land-locked creatures in the entire history of the earth! They are about to see the world from a perspective unlike any that their slippery 'froggy' kin had ever seen. The bad news was that they will more than likely pay a very heavy price for the privilege; that price being the ultimate; death."

Wow! As a young teenager I was getting excited. Dad was a great teacher but I must admit, he did seem to have a rather weird 'mean' streak in him.

He then sat straight up and took aim. He pulled the trigger and with a thunderous boom the can shuddered and the water contained in the can, along with its amphibious occupants, exploded upwards out of the can and into the sky above.

The frogs, no-doubt by now somewhat dazed at the least, were still intact and with arms and legs extended they were in a state of suspended animation high in the air, very high indeed above the Salmon River, getting a view of that part of the world that, like Dad had said, no other frog had ever, ever seen! Awesome I thought.

The frogs, dead or alive, were never to be seen by my eyes again but the image of them high in the sky over the river did in fact leave an indelible impression in my brain.

Let's fast-forward and get back to my medical career. In the mid-80s I had vague knowledge and cursory interest in lithotripters which were the emerging non-invasive medical devices that break up kidney stones. My interest like I said was there but nowhere near strong enough to really motivate me to dig deeper into the technology.

All that was about to change in 1993 when I was invited by Pat Varan and some other folks at Siemens to put my creative strategic marketing expertise to work for them regarding a very revolutionary new lithotripter that they were developing.

It was really a fascinating machine, in that it was the first to effectively disintegrate kidney stones utilizing an 'optimized-pressure' system that operated well under the threshold of tissue destruction; very, very different from the other high-pressure units out there. The clinical benefits were huge; the fact that it operated below tissue-destroying force meant that it was painless thus eliminating the need for anesthesia; the patient could actually 'work with you' during therapy!

It also utilized a 3-dimensional X-Ray 'stone' locating system allowing for the 'in situ' treatment of Ureteral stones; Ureteral stones representing about 30% of all urinary tract stones.

Unlike the High-Pressure units there would be no loss of blood, no loss of bladder control, no effect on sexual ability and no anesthesia leaving the patient fully awake and aware and able to resume normal activities within an hour of the normal 30 to 45 minute treatment.

I was impressed and it was not long before I accepted the challenge from Siemens to personally introduce and integrate this technology into the mainstream managed care communities in the United States.

We had come a long way indeed from when my Mother had her kidney stones!

What is ESWL and how does it work?

Extracorporeal Shock Wave Lithotripsy (ESWL) is a technology used to treat Kidney and Ureteral stones as well as Bladder and Gall stones. Extracorporeal means outside of the body and the word Lithotripsy is derived from the Greek words 'tripto' which means to 'crush' and 'litho' meaning stone.

The human anatomy is made up mostly of hydrogen. It was discovered that one could generate an external force and transfer that force into the body with absolute minimal loss of this destructive force. ESWL works by delivering externally created 'targeted' shockwaves into the human anatomy where they destroy the 'targeted' stones.

ESWL was introduced in the late 1970s and has undergone many developmental and technical changes over the years, however, the underlying physics has remained the same.

There are two basic categories of lithotripters available today; the older High-Pressure type and the newer Optimized Low-Pressure variety.

I had been working with a number of prominent urologists as a consultant in a deal where they were providing mobile lithotripsy services to outlying hospitals. They were all utilizing the heavy duty Dornier HM3 'Big Bangers' that required that the patients be fully anesthetized and submerged in a large water bath; in reality a cauldron containing a huge spark plug in the bottom.

The 'Big Banger' worked in a rather archaic, torturous manner, however, it did work, but because of its quasi-controllable destructive powers, only on calculi (stones) actually located in the kidneys.

This presented one of my first serious dilemmas regarding this unit; the fact that it could not be used for ureteral stones was definitely problematic. When I asked the urologists about this their normal answer was that they would insert a stent (a small flexible tube) into the patient's ureter (the tube connecting the kidneys and the bladder) as soon as possible to stop the stone from moving, then as soon as was feasible (convenient?) they would physically manipulate the obstacle back into the kidney where they could then use the high-pressure 'Big Banger' to blast the stone into smaller, more manageable pieces.

As a result of the intra-kidney pressures somewhere in the 1000/lb per sq. in. range the actual procedure with the Dornier lithotripter it was not unusual for the patient to suffer substantial kidney and surrounding tissue damage, blood loss, temporary loss of bladder control, temporary erectile dysfunction as well as the need for weeks of recuperation.

There was little doubt in my mind that the Siemens optimized-pressure unit was a superior technology that, if used properly could provide significant positive benefits and patient outcomes regarding kidney stone treatments; not to mention the ability to eliminate the questionable 'stenting' procedure altogether!

I conferred with the VP of Blue Cross and Blue Shield of Central Florida regarding my proposed plan to provide BC&BS superior urolithiasis treatments at a fraction of their global treatment costs. He agreed to hear me out. I also had made myself aware of the legal and technical requirements of BC&BS that governed their ability to contract with private health care firms.

I had enlisted a very well respected urologist who was an actual member of the FDA onto my team as my Medical Director so I would be well represented on the clinical side. I then carefully pieced together my version of the kidney stone treatment 'Ben Franklin Balance Sheet' and ultimately headed off to see Dr. Joe and the BC&BS clinical executive Board.

Dr. Joe and his colleagues were very tough but very fair. They listened to my pitch, carefully weighed the rather voluminous clinical and research data and within a few months and many, many meetings the Board agreed; it was a no-brainer. We had a deal; the very first contract with managed care for *mandated* low-pressure lithotripsy in the State of Florida at a global cost of $3,200 per patient as opposed to the $16,000 global fee that they had been paying.

Anesthesia-free treatments, no loss of blood or bladder control, no erectile function problems, the ability to treat ureteral stones and the elimination of the whole stenting procedure and its resultant risks and costs. Far better clinical outcomes at a fraction of the cost; what more could you want?

Over the next few months we built a world-class lithotripsy center and were in business; BC&BS contract in hand. Our center was the first in the world to treat not only without anesthesia; we did not even use the common pre-treatment analgesia. We had developed a protocol whereby we would apply a freeze pack directly to the site where the shock tube would contact the patient. That, combined with headphones and the patient's favorite music eliminated the need for any pre-treatment patient prep.

It was common sense that brought about the myriad of questions by managed care regarding stenting. Common sense dictated that if in fact the offending stone had left the kidney and made its way down the ureter that, if left alone and the patient were given effective analgesia and over-hydration, the stone would most likely exit on its own.

Our research clearly illustrated that stenting the patient, in all but the most unusual of circumstances, was absolutely not necessary. Worse case would be that the stone did not move at which point the patient could be treated in a clinically-timely manner as a result of the lack of need for preparation and anesthesia. All was great; well, not exactly!

"Regrettably even the greatest of urology specialists are not immune to Urolithiasis nor, even more regrettably, are they immune to 'ethical challenge'!"

Did I mention that most, actually all of the lithotripters in the US were owned by the various urology groups across the nation. Virtually all of the urologists in Florida either owned or were directly involved as partners in for-profit lithotripsy programs and as a result were making substantial amounts of money from them. When we got involved virtually all of the lithotripters were Dornier HM3 Big Bangers. And here we come, an optimized-pressure lithotripsy organization headed up by me, a non-urologist with a contract from BC&BS mandating that all of their group urologists utilize our, yes our new optimized-pressure lithotripter service!

We had invaded their world and, needless to say, the natives were getting pretty restless! The urologists did not take lightly to the BC&BS mandate that their stone patients had to be treated at our low-pressure litho center.

Again I reflect back to my good friend Carter and ask that we follow the 'bouncing dollar bill'. Why would an intelligent professional, in this case a urologist who has taken the Hippocratic Oath, subject his patient to a far more risky, less effective treatment that required general anesthesia and most likely stenting when a far less risky, more effective treatment requiring no anesthesia, no analgesia and no stenting was readily available?

I asked that question far too many times and BC&BS did also. The answer, unfortunately, was obvious; the urologists were willing to forego patient safety and comfort for the sole benefit of their pockets.... Money. They made far more money with their 'Big Bangers' than they could with the safer, more effective optimized-pressure Siemens Lithostar.

Ethical challenge often-times has no bounds; both I and Dr. Joe experienced everything from having my Cadillac acid-bathed at the obvious hands of a disgruntled physician, law suits and restraining orders through to actual death threats against us!

When it came to many of the local urologists and their choice between making money and the Hippocratic Oath you can guess what came out ahead; just follow the bouncing dollars! In perhaps the greatest display of group ethical challenge the regional urologists actually 'yanked' their professional services from BC&BS and, unfortunately, their patients. They actually refused to provide any post-treatment care to any patient that came to our facility; they would not see that patient regardless of whether it was treatment related or not.

"The operation was a success but, unfortunately, the patient died!"

It was a very taxing time indeed and one which presented me and Dr. Joe with our own ethical dilemma; do we 'aid and abet' the urologists in their quasi-legal, totally unethical stance or do we restore sanity into the system by giving them access to what they really wanted, not the new, more effective technology but the money stream coming from our center!

Their blackmail tactics worked and we 'caved in' turning the company and its centers over to the urologists who, not surprisingly, quickly closed the doors. They went back to their old ways of processing their patients with the 'Big Bangers' and willingly providing post-treatment care to all who had been traumatized in the procedure.

Even today, decades later, many urologists are still subjecting their patients to the older Dornier units and the resultant kidney and bladder damage. Why? The 'Cash Cow' is still pooping big dollars! Even those urologists who have reluctantly converted to the newer, optimized-pressure lithotripters are still subjecting their 'stone' patients to anesthesia and most are back to actually 'stenting' the patient as well!

The whole reason for optimized-pressure lithotripsy was and remains to be able to treat below the threshold of tissue destruction and pain, thus eliminating the need for anesthesia. The other primary reason is the ability to treat ureteral stones without having to manipulate the stone at all; there is no need for a stent!

What motivates the urologists to do so; I hate to be the one to tell you the truth but it is MONEY; pure and simple.

Medical Tip:
If you or a family member suffers a kidney stone attack, please use your God given common sense when it comes to accepting your good doctor's recommendations. If he doesn't recommend a low-pressure unit move on quickly and find another that will.

> *"Let's again remember the TITANIC was built by experts!"*

The engineers for Siemens responsible for site acceptability had shown up to inspect the building where we were going to open the center. It was on the 3rd floor of a rather posh office building adjacent to a major hospital on the outskirts of Orlando. We were well on our way as we had been working off of a set of preliminary plans that had been prepared for us by Siemens on the site for a month or so. We had the walls up, some of the plumbing and most of the overhead electrical conduits for cables already in place according to the original drawings.

One of the engineers came into what was to be the actual 'litho' room and unfolded another set of drawings on the work table. He motioned me over and pointed up where we had three 40 feet long, 2" conduits installed.

"All that has to be changed," he said pointing to the conduits, "according to these new plans you need 12" conduits not those 2 inchers."

He was the expert, after all, and after much discussion he convinced us that we absolutely needed to remove the much lighter 2" conduits and replace them with much, much heavier 12" ones. I had the architect review the new requirements and he said that we would have to reinforce the complete overhead building structure to accommodate the significantly heavier steel conduits at a very, very significant cost..

I went back and forth with Siemens regarding this 'oversight' of theirs but to no avail; we went ahead, bit the financial bullet and made the required changes to the building to accommodate the larger 12" pipes. A couple of weeks of serious reconstruction flew by and it was finally time to open the wooden crates and extract and install the equipment.

I remember as the electrician was running the cables through the 12" conduits in the ceiling he asked,
"Why in the hell did you use 12" conduits?"
"Siemens instructed us to, They said that the cables had 11.5" connectors on them which had to be threaded through the conduits."
"Are you sure we have the right cables?" he replied "the fittings on these things are only about one and a half inches."
Everything came to a screeching halt as I got Siemens on the line.

We had the right cables alright and the actual fittings were only one and a half inches across; the foam shipping protectors, which you were instructed to remove before threading the cables into the conduits, were in fact 11.5" in diameter!

Just that one fiasco cost us close to one hundred thousand dollars!

And don't think that the clinical treatment side of new medical technologies is immune to fiascos; it most assuredly is not!

It was a big day for Lithotripsy in Florida; we had our first actual non-research kidney stone patient on the table and we were ready to go. The treatment pressure tube had risen from the table and was in place separated from the patient only by a thin layer of 'gel' that came from Siemens with the lithotripter.

The top clinical executives from BC&BS were in the observation room along with Pat Varan and another exec from Siemens. The patient had his headphones on and was grooving away to his 'tunes' totally oblivious to what was going on in the control room.

Our Medical Director had set the treatment parameters on the console and anxiously pressed the Start button; the soft clicking sounds started indicating that the pressure tubes had been activated and therapy was in fact underway.

A 'normal' treatment would last about thirty or forty minutes and, like flying or sailing, should be uneventful; bordering on boring! The BC&BS people sat there transfixed on the patient; watching what can best be described as the medical treatment version of watching paint dry!

I was in the control room with my Medical Director actually joking about something unrelated to the treatment when I noticed the 'gel' had gone from clear to a definite pinkish hue; something that I had never seen in all of our research. I pointed this out to the Medical Director who was also somewhat perplexed at the color transition. We discussed the possibilities and came to the conclusion that the reason for the pinkish hue was most likely the astonishing addition of blood to the gel; something that should not be possible with low-pressure lithotripsy.

Because of the fact that the execs from BC&BS were watching what was going on we most certainly did not want to spook them; we decided that we would just sort of saunter over to the table to get a closer look before we panicked. We really knew what was happening but just did not want to acknowledge it.

The short version of this story was that it was indeed blood. We had somehow poked a hole in this guy about the size of a pencil and about two inches deep!

We pulled the covers over the patients bleeding mid-section and shut the unit down. We told the BC&BS execs that we had to reposition the patient and restart the treatment. Fortunately they had prior commitments and had to leave. Within minutes the patient was resting comfortably next door in the hospital.

Siemens subsequently had somehow settled with the patient without any publicity; thank goodness; we were still alive!

What happened was that Siemens had shipped Ultrasound gel with our Lithostar, not the required purer, de-gassed litho gel. As their scientists sort of explained the minuscule bubbles in the Ultrasound gel actually magnified the intensity of the shockwaves and somehow, miraculously destroyed the tissue in its path!

Isn't technology awesome!

CHAPTER SEVEN
COMMON SENSE AND DISEASE MANAGEMENT & PREVENTION

" Common sense often drowns in the calm sea of education!"

Whenever I get asked to describe what common sense is I am reminded that the answer to that is sort of like pornography; it's hard to explain what it is but you will know it when you see it!

The easiest way for me to explain what common sense is to clearly illustrate what it is not.

Arthur A. Jones was the inventor of the Nautilus exercise equipment. Arthur was a rough, tough guy who lived life to extreme excess, smoked like a chimney and died of natural causes at 80. He was also an avid lover of very, very dangerous animals; perhaps that is why he had six wives!

I remember hearing him relate a story about a trip he took to Africa to film a documentary on Hippopotamus, the most feared of all wild African beasts. There was one particular lake that the locals avoided because of the danger imposed by the large population of hippos. He and his crew hired a guide with a team of well armed locals just in case. They had all piled into a truck and off they went to the lake. Upon arriving at the lake they saw another truck and four or five people who seemed to be Americans. This group of people were putting on their swimming attire. Arthur got out of the truck.
"Excuse me but what in the hell do you think you are doing?"
"It's hotter than hell; we're going swimming."
"Do you realize that there are dozens of hippos in there? You people really should not be here."
"Oh, that's OK" was the reply, "we're with the Peace Corps"!

That is *definitely* what common sense is NOT!

When we look at common sense and how it plays into personally preventing most deadly diseases the picture gets pretty murky. What we do know is that worrying about it definitely does not help. And the 'experts', whoever-the-hell they are, also don't help. If you really want to worry yourself 'stupid' just look at any list of risk factors compiled by these so-called experts; there is plenty of fodder for worry-warts! There are more than 200 of risk factors just for Coronary Artery Disease ranging from Family History, Blood Pressure and Lifestyle to C-Reative Protein, Homocystein, HDL and LDL levels; like I said it will truly drive you nuts!

My answer to all this is to just relax; use your God given common sense and do your own assessment. It is like voting; do it early and do it often!

Let's look at Blood Pressure. A huge percentage of the population that see their doctor are on blood pressure regulating medication. I will be the first to admit that Blood Pressure is most likely a very meaningful indicator of something, maybe CAD, if you are looking at large populations, however, when it comes to BP as a precursor of CAD in individuals the correlation is not so clear at all. Lets you and I again reflect upon my own personal experience with BP.

I am 70 plus years of age; on absolutely no medication and I am doing what appears to be very well indeed walking up and down a 2500 foot driveway with a 200 foot elevation change, and doing it twice daily!

The first time it was very strongly recommended by a cardiologist that I get on BP regulation was some 40 years ago. After looking into the side effects, especially the longer-term ones, my common sense told me to 'just say no' and to start being extra vigilant for other indications of impending trouble; then maybe do something.

Ever since I first started racing motorcycles in the 70s my normal 'first' BP reading has been in the 210 over 160 range; Death City! Most cardiologists that have taken my BP simply lay me down on their couch and go to another room and call an ambulance; no kidding; they all think that I am going to 'explode' right there in their office.

After a few more readings my BP usually will be down to a far more so-called 'normal' range; in the 130/90.

I tell you this because again I assert that risk factors are great for dealing with huge populations but all but useless when dealing with individuals.

There are two main problems in dealing with disease in this country, especially coronary artery disease;

1. Our inability to properly assess an individual's risk of disease.
2. Our inability to properly assess an individual's actual response to therapy for the disease.

The simple answer to this very complex problem is to just fix these two obvious shortfalls in our clinical processes. The resultant positive patient outcomes would pretty well eradicate most serious diseases in a very timely fashion.

If all of these risk factors, especially BP were indeed a truly accurate indicator of impending serious medical consequences you would not be reading this book; it would have never been written; I would have blown apart in some poor cardiologist's office or in the ambulance that they had summoned... I WOULD BE DEAD! If I were to inject the other risk factors on top of hyper-elevated BP into my personal mix, hell, I would really be DEAD; in fact I would be DOUBLE DEAD if that is possible.

Maybe the worry-warts are right and the real answer to a long, healthy life is to actually agonize over every little thing that happens, and more importantly, can happen to you.

Worry, worry and then worry some more; after all, in all actuality you most probably do have ample legitimate reasons to do so, however, I hate to be the bearer of bad news here but there is little, if any, legitimate research illustrating any real genuine benefits of doing so.

Maybe, just maybe the old adage of 'when your time is up; your time is up' is just the plain, unadulterated truth and something that we should just 'go' with.

FOOD FOR THOUGHT:

Story 1.

I had a good entrepreneurial friend in Montreal who at the age of 45 had survived a massive heart attack. He was taken to one of the major hospitals downtown where he ultimately stayed for months of cardiac rehab.

During his hospitalization his wife took over in the business and was actually quite adept at running a mid-size enterprise. The day finally came when his cardiologist declared him ready to go home. Tim was quite anxious to get beck home and one step closer to getting back to his work. He was overjoyed and far beyond optimistic about his future, almost feeling invincible; after all he had survived what normally kills all of its victims.

He called his wife and informed her of the doctor's decision; she was also elated but somewhat apprehensive as she was now fully involved in the business and could not supply the essential care needed. They agreed that all would work out and that they would just have to take it one day at a time.

His wife went by the hospital that night and collected all of his personal belongings. She explained that there was a very important, long-scheduled business meeting the following day and that they simply could not afford to forego. All that Tim had to do was to get his discharge papers out of the way then go out front and take a taxi home.

Like I stated the hospital was right downtown and built on a boulevard that was six lanes separated by a 20 or so foot median. The cardiologist signed Tim's discharge papers, gave him some prescriptions and, as they rolled Tim to the front entrance in the mandatory wheelchair, wished Tim well at the doors.

Tim got out of the chair, shook the doc's hand and joyfully walked through the hospital's large doors clutching his precious discharge papers. He walked to the edge of the street and tried to flag a taxi down. His first two attempts went unanswered, however, he saw a cab approaching in the opposite direction on the outside lanes. He again flailed his arms in the air and to his relief the cab pulled over and stopped to wait for him to cross the street. Tim, I suspect, was overanxious to get home and in his haste to do so stepped from the sidewalk into the street.

Tim was struck by a bus and passed away on the street mere feet away from the hospital that he had just left.

Story 2.

I had another close friend in Central Florida who also survived a massive heart attack and was also hospitalized for an extended period of time.

After months of rehab he was discharged. He heeded all of the advice of his cardiologist and underwent a dramatic life style change, including trading in his Harley Davidson motorcycle for a very serious looking road racing bicycle.

Rick was not only a friend but also a neighbor of mine living down the street from me in a great upscale community just north of Orlando. There were a lot of physical fitness fanatics in the community so it did not take long for Rick to hook up with a number of them who were into long distance bike rides on the weekends; the perfect match for him and his goals of getting and staying in top physical condition to avoid another heart attack.

The first ride was a Sunday outing that would take them from Longwood to New Smyrna Beach and back, a total distance of seventy miles or so.

It was fall in Central Florida and the weather was absolutely perfect; 70 some degrees and crystal clear skies as the group headed out. They had made it about three-quarters of the way to the beach when a car ran a stop sign and plowed into one of the cyclists.

Rick was in the absolute best shape of his life, however, fate took over and he died at the scene.

Rick was a very healthy 48 years young but a very dead 48!

Now, you may think that the moral of these two stories is that you should never, ever, under any circumstances, become a close friend of mine. That is not my motive for relating these stories. The moral being asserted here is that you can worry yourself stupid about your health but you really have little control over what cards will be dealt to you in life that will end your game.

Common sense DIY diagnostic and disease preventative studies that you can do at home.

There are many things that you can do on your own; simple tests that you can perform on yourself to see if you have any indications of disease or if you are declining in health in any number of areas.
Cardiovascular:

Because this is the number one killer of mankind I suggest that you first find out whether in fact you have heart disease before you go on any medication for this disease **or any of its symptoms!**

"The best indication of cardiovascular Disease is actual evidence of Cardiovascular Disease."

*Get a CT Calcium study before anything else; the presence of calcium (CA) in your arteries means that you definitely have the disease!!!

*Every morning when you are 'on the pot' take a pin and prick the tip of each and every toe. You will quickly detect any loss of feeling meaning a possible circulatory problem.

Eyes:
Here is a good question:
Why is it when you go to the ophthalmologist and get a new prescription for either glasses or contacts and you go to get it filled it takes a week or so to get them, however, when you need a replacement you can show up at any Eyeglass Superstore and get them in an hour! Does every single Eyeglass Superstore keep a supply of your personal prescription lenses in stock or is the initial delay some kind of conspiracy to justify the initial costs?

What can you do at home?
*Get an eye chart; you know the chart that the eye doctors use to test your vision. They may be hard to find because

the ophthalmologists really do not want you to have one. I suspect that they buy up and destroy as many old eye charts as they can find to stop you from getting one!

*Once you get an eye chart put it up somewhere where you can test yourself under the same conditions weekly. Take detailed notes; you will soon see if something is wrong. Your eyes are muscles and like all other muscles in your body they require regular exercise. The process of testing yourself will be a great exercise for your eyes.

I was prescribed glasses when I was thirteen and wore them until sixteen or so when I started playing contact (no pun intended) sports. I kept breaking my glasses and simply gave up wearing them. As a result I was forced to squint and forcefully adjust my eyes to see what I had to; in other words I was unintentionally exercising my eyes. I am going on 71 and have not worn glasses or contacts since sixteen and my eyesight is absolutely superb; I can see a fly 'taking a dump' a hundred feet away!

Do your own 'Field of Vision' Study:
*Stand up straight and focus on a spot directly in front of you; perhaps your eye chart. Extend your arms out fully from your sides and move your fingers. If you don't see them start bringing your arms forward until you can. Take detailed notes of these angles as if it were a clock; 3 to noon on the right and 9 to noon on the left. Do the same above and below your head. Repeat this process every month and compare the results to see if there are any changes. If there is any reduction in what you see then go to your ophthalmologist.

Ears:
*Get a set of good ear bud headphones, some good earplugs and some music that you like. Turn off all noise making devices as possible. Insert the ear bud into the right ear and insert a plug in the left ear. Turn on the music but turn the volume to zero. Now increase the volume one click at a time until you just start hearing the music. Again, take detailed notes. Now do the same for the right ear and take notes. Do

this test every 3 months and compare the results.
*Check your stool (not what you are sitting on at a bar!) and urine daily for blood, puss, albumen or any other unusual or foreign looking substances. I know, I know but just do it OK!

Just Use Your Common Sense! Don't smoke; don't drink; don't eat red meat, actually don't eat any meat; stay away from eggs; only eat gluten-free bread; stay out of the sun, actually don't even go outside; stay away from automobiles, buses, motorcycles, scooters, trucks and motor boats; the exhaust you know!

Don't glare at your computer screen or TV; keep your cell phone away from your head; don't breathe second-hand anything; use face masks whenever you do dare to venture out; stay the hell away from the backside of cows; do not wander out onto a street for any reason; shellfish are taboo; do not sleep on any motel or hotel bed; and definitely do not breathe the air in an airplane, in fact don't ever fly; the closer to the sun the higher the radiation levels!

Just follow the above rules and you may just outlive everyone; especially all of your friends who actually enjoyed life and what it had to offer them.

My father told me a joke when I was just a young lad. It stuck with me and is a very appropriate way for me to end this book.

There was a man from Boston who was absolutely terrified of flying. His job required that he attend a very important meeting in Miami. Given his fear of flying he decided to take the train and enjoy a wonderful stress-free ride down the East coast of the country. He died in North Carolina when a plane crashed into the train!

"Don't worry; be happy" as the song from the seventies suggests we all do.

Most likely inherited from father
my personal maxim has always been;
"I'm willing to check out of the hotel early as long as I get to the party the night before!"

CHAPTER EIGHT
WANES, WESSELS, PLUCK AND WHO IN HELL IS PERRY FERREL?

I recall back in the late 70s being the guest speaker at a meeting of the Canadian Nursing Association in Ottawa, Canada's capital city. During my talk, one doctor in the audience bellowed out "There's nothing funny about death Mr. Mueller, nothing funny at all." While that may be true about death itself, there are often times that comedic relief can be discovered in the circumstances surrounding death. This doc's outburst resulted from the fact that in the midst of what was in fact a very serious message regarding the psychological woes of caring for the dying I had somehow managed to bring up the death of 'Chuckles' the Clown on the then favorite Mary Tyler Moore TV show. I had brought Chuckles up in an attempt to convey a message that, even when you are dealing in the most serious of situations, you must not let it get the best of you and comedy is more often than not the best relief. Now, lest you have forgotten, let's get back to poor Chuckles. Any true aficionado of the TV show, as most Americans were, must remember "A little song, a little dance, a little seltzer in your pants"; don't you? Surely you haven't forgotten how Chuckles died. Let's digress for a moment and take advantage of this great opportunity to test out my theory regarding comedic relief, here and now.

Close your eyes and think of someone who you loved dearly, someone who has recently passed away. Are you feeling sad yet, hopefully you are getting very, very sad; emotionally unstable, in fact it will be best if you are actually tearing up a bit. Okay, now that you are fully engaged in the pre-depression blues let me proceed with the story. Do you remember just how Chuckles died? He actually went out in a big way. Chuckles in fact met his untimely demise as the Grand Marshal in a circus parade where he was dressed as Peter Peanut. During the procession a rogue parade elephant broke loose, grabbed poor Peter and tried to "shell" him; he died from his injuries. Geez, now that I think about it, maybe there is nothing funny about death, or this story.

In all honesty I really feel that the good vocal doctor was wrong and the 'Chuckles' thing proved it; other than him the rest of the audience in Ottawa were chuckling, no pun intended. They were actually doing so quite loudly; so it must have worked. I truly believe that there is humor to be found in just about everything but more often than not you must seek it out. Another great example of this occurred one day a few years back when I switched on the TV and my usual cable news network came on. You could tell immediately that they were televising a funeral, and quite a large one at that. It was a terribly dreary day; probably if one had a choice, the perfect day for a funeral. From the size of the crowd and the fact that it was being televised I suspected that it was a State funeral for a dignitary or perhaps an entertainment celebrity of some sorts. The broadcasters were very, very good, in that they made you feel as though you personally had just lost your mother and father along with all of your family in a terrible and very excruciatingly painful accident. I can still hear the announcer saying, in a very somber tone "it is a very sad day indeed; dreary, drizzling, cold but it will all be just a memory soon." There was the typical wide shot of the area as he continued, "And to think that this man's life will be forever reduced to this scene is unbelievably sad in itself," he continued, "the last vision of this man that most of you in the audience will have is that of the Honor Guard placing the casket into the back of that big beautiful gray horse!" Wow, now that is the way to go; never mind the hearse, just stick me in the rear-end of a horse! You could hear all involved in the broadcast roaring in the background. See, I was right; there is humor to be found in just about everything, even funerals.

On a more personal note. Many years ago the mother of one of my brother-in-laws had passed away. She really was a fine woman whose name was Lucille. I personally liked her very, very much and felt a great personal loss at her passing. The entire extended family attended the funeral. It was truly a sad event, as I said she was a very nice and likeable person. Immediately after the traditional lowering of the casket we headed for our cars. The funeral had been held in a somewhat remote area with only a few radio stations available. My brother started his car. He had his radio set at its normal volume which was rather high at which point the sound started blaring from his car and the song that was playing was Kenny Rogers' "You picked a fine time to leave me Lucille". It brought more than a few laughs to the grieving crowd; timing is everything.

You may have to look long and hard to find humor but, low-and-behold, it will be there somewhere, perhaps hidden by even more tragedy, death or mayhem. A good, highly polished sense of humor will definitely help as well. Sometimes, especially in foreign countries with language barriers, humor is in the translations surrounding mayhem. In Germany, even though a 'sense of humor' is a rare find indeed, humorous situations surrounding the misfortunes of others are really not hard to find. The Germans, in fact, have their own word for this exact thing! Meine güte (my gosh), am I glad to be of German heritage, that's probably where my weird sense of humor came from. *Schadenfreude* is their word and it means (and *mean* it is!) *satisfaction or pleasure felt at someone else's misfortune!* The word is derived from the German words *schaden* meaning harm and *freude* meaning joy. Ach du lieber! (Oh heavens!), what a funny place The Faderland is, just chocked full of funny people; not too many comedy clubs though.

Schadenfreude is everywhere to be found in Germany; especially if you are a tourist, however, it will be you that will most likely be on the receiving end of the schaden, while they take unbelievable pleasure in the joys of the freude, at your personal expense! Not all is bad, however, because I can assure you that schadenfreude changes dramatically if you are a cardiovascular imaging executive and have been given unfettered access to their medical facilities. In that case you will get to roam freely within their cardiac clinics and see first-hand the rather rotund German mountain men in their unbelievably multi-colored, wacky, overly-revealing 'undies'. Oh, here we go off on a tangent. I once took a group of cardiologists from Columbia, SC to Germany for a first-hand assessment of the clinical benefits of a new cardiac imaging technology. After days and days of intense research and patient studies at the famous Klinikum Grosshadern in Munich we had come to the end of the project. I gathered them around the CT scanner in the cardiac unit and asked if there were any questions that they had that had not been answered. One of them looked at me and said, "The only question I have is where in the hell do the men get those huge, skimpy, weird T-backs?" So much for clinical research. Unglaublich, Ach du lieber, erneut! (unbelievable, oh heavens again!) But oh how I digress.

To fully appreciate the rest of the story I must set the stage and take you back in time to when I first got involved in, and with, the global cardiovascular community.

I was in my mid-fifties, full of energy and I was pretty excited at my personal breakthrough. Here I was, a non-cardiologist, in fact not even a physician, and I had just been contracted with one of the major global medical technology manufacturers to 'lead the charge' in the development of a strategic program for the education, introduction and systematic integration surrounding a new cardiovascular imaging technology into the global mainstream healthcare delivery systems.

Just so that your mind does not go too far astray, I was not totally ill-equipped for this lofty position. I had owned and operated a number of cardiovascular imaging centers over the years and had been acknowledged as an 'expert in the field' by a number of States in the clinical utilization of CT in cardiovascular disease management. I need not go fully into the sordid details of how this came about, sort of like Chance, the gardener in the Peter Sellers movie 'Being There', I sort of fell into this awesome gig; one of those right place at the right time type of deals. The fact that I was not even a physician, let alone a cardiologist, was never even a factor. My lack of medical credentials had taken a back seat to the desire for profits out of a new marketplace by the Board of Directors of the company. My non-physician status was overshadowed by my most unique, and I do mean unique, combination of a strong knowledge of the clinical processes involving cardiovascular disease, an innate understanding of the physics and mechanics of the emerging technology and its applicability to the detection, identification and quantification of Coronary Artery Disease (CAD), coupled with my personal acceptability and, of course, my ability to communicate complex concepts and theories in simple, down-to-earth terms; you know, the 'Chuckles the Clown' thing. I really understood how this technology worked and exactly how it could impact Coronary Artery Disease rates if it were utilized properly upon the proper selection of people suspected of having the number one killing disease. I considered this contract not in terms of an income but more of a mission, a global one at that, and on the mission I was.

Although I was working mainly out of the American head office in New Jersey, I was actually contracted with the global nerve center and headquarters of the corporation in Nurnberg, Germany. With that, much to the chagrin of my chief supporter, my wife, came offices in Nurnberg and Munich, Germany in addition to my office in Orlando and Philadelphia. As Oscar Wilde would have said "the good news is that I had offices in Germany; the bad news is that I had offices in Germany!" As a consequence of this I had to be seen in these German offices occasionally if for no other reason than to show that I was still alive and kicking and worthy of the somewhat generous checks that I was receiving. My schedule was truly grueling involving far too many cross-country and International flights with far too little time to relax anywhere, including home. To say that my duties were diverse would be a gross understatement. A large part of my responsibilities was to engage those experts at all levels of clinical practice and research regarding CAD. I was to immerse myself in not only my work, but also in their clinical efforts so that I could fully assess the marketplace and, armed with that knowledge, work directly with the corporate physicists to develop new applications and sort of 'hone' the technology to better address what I saw as the needs of the cardiology community.

Immerse myself I did and in short order there I was, Herr Mueller, in attendance as an invited guest to address the American cardiology community at a meeting in San Francisco regarding this emerging technology and how it could be used in our common quest to eradicate heart attacks. Since most of the research for clinical validation of the technology had taken place at a number of major medical centers in Europe, there were a number of the European research cardiologists in attendance as well. I had already 'bonded' with a number of these foreign experts on prior trips to Europe so they were comfortable in comparing notes and sharing thoughts with me regarding our presentations and the technology itself. At the end of the meeting one of the cardiologists from the University of Heidelberg offered me a personal invitation to participate in a meeting about CAD being held at the University two weeks later. I willingly accepted.

The flight to Heidelberg, actually to Frankfurt with another fight to Heidelberg was the all-too-familiar red-eye where I would leave my home in the mid morning and get to New York in the afternoon, make a few visits to the local cardiac units and leave for Europe mid evening. That way I would get to my destination in Germany in the early hours of the next morning, just in time for a whole extra long day's work. Well, anyway I made it to Heidelberg (my luggage did not!) and the meeting convened at noon and we were off and at it; truly on the mission. Now, as you can well imagine, the subject matter and clinical research details are dry, and I mean dry. "There is nothing funny about CAD research, Doctors!" I was often tempted to scream out, not from any attempts at humor being displayed but the subject matter was so dry, except for the blood of course, and it just went on and on. I had, however, willingly volunteered for this gig, so there I sat taking copious notes and trying to decipher the ultra-complex clinical content of the talks while viewing colored slides of every possible anomalous growth and gross pathology associated with the fist-sized organ we call the heart. Lest I forget I must also add that English is the universal language at cardiology conventions. I will give you a clue; look for the use of the word humor coming up soon. Alright, not only was I tasked with figuring out the clinical implications of the masses, blobs, dissections and other abundant pathological disorders being displayed in full, blood-dripping color but I was also trying to figure out what the hell they were actually saying in their attempt to deliver their talks in English. Being sleep-deprived did not help one bit. To offset my inability to fully grasp what was really going on with the 'spoken word' I just kept taking notes, lots and lots of notes, some in a simplified phonetic form for me to try and make sense of later on, when I could really concentrate on the content. "Maybe a good shot or three of Scotch will help" is what I would tell myself.

After we had finished for the day I went to my hotel and freshened up. I then went out for dinner. I took the leisurely stroll that the locals suggested which was a two mile winding trek up a very narrow cobblestone pathway pretty well directly up the side of the mountain to the plateau upon which the famous castle in Heidelberg sits high above the city majestically overlooking the Neckar River. I had dinner in the castle's main dining room; it was a magnificent way to spend the evening. Walking back down the meandering roadway in the dark was easier than going up, however, the ingestion of more than adequate amounts of wine at dinner added a new and somewhat dangerous element into the mix. After an hour or so of wondering aimlessly like a stray dog around the city of Heidelberg I finally found my way back to the hotel.

I showered and got ready for bed. I sat down on the couch and grabbed my notes from the conference. I had pages and pages of detailed notes about hematomas, arterial dissections, bifurcation involving calcification, aortic root tumors, sub-pericardial hemorrhaging, wow, I couldn't help but wonder how any of us are still breathing!

Although my notes were detailed there were many, many

places where they were not coherent, they simply didn't make sense. I had numerous arrows off to the sides of the pages where, even more confusing, were the phonetic words "wanes, wessels and pluck" that I had repeatedly scribbled. I recalled questioning these words at the conference because they just kept coming up over and over again and by multiple speakers, in fact pretty well all of the presenters were commenting regarding these wanes, wessels and pluck. Tired and more than a little inebriated I really could not make sense of it; I put the notes down and went into the bedroom.

With the normal imaginary conference-attending chest pain setting in, I got into bed wondering just how long it would take me to die from some form of excruciating aortic explosion or other life ending hemo-redirecting event. Asleep I fell but not for long. I woke up about an hour later, sat up in the bed and said to myself, "you butthole! They are saying veins, vessels and plaque!" How stupid could I get? It really should have been obvious to me but, like I said, I aint no cardiologist and it was not exactly a Berlitz language course going on there! At least now more of my notes from the day should make more sense. Again there really is humor in almost all situations. Laughing at my stupidity and smiling like a mad dog I lay back down and went back to sleep.

I awoke at daybreak, rested and raring to go. I showered and dressed and went out on the terrace for breakfast. I was staying at the Marriott directly on the banks of the Neckar River. It was marvelous as the sun was just coming up and the city was just starting to come alive for yet another wonderful day in a truly wonderful city.

The conference started at 8:00 sharp, so off I went, notebooks in hand, for the final day of the formal meetings. After another humorless session just chocked full of full-colored stomach-churning pathological anomalies lunch was in order. I sat down with the chief cardiologist from the University Hospital. We of course started talking about the meeting and how wonderful it was to have such a gathering of experts all dedicated to the furtherance of this marvelous technology.

"Dr. Hilldenberg" I said, "if you look a couple of years into the future what do you see happening with this technology?"

With little hesitation he looked at me and said "Herr Mueller, the answer is with Perry Ferrel; Perry Ferrel is without doubt the future of this technology."

I had been involved in cardiovascular CT for quite a while at that point and had never even heard of this guy. It bothered me a bit since it was my primary responsibility to be in touch with anyone and everyone in the know regarding cardiovascular CT. Who in the hell was this Perry Ferrel?

"Is Perry Ferrel here at the conference?" I asked

He glanced at me in that *are you really that stupid?* Look. "No, that would have been too confusing for the others," he said; he just continued eating.

Wanting to find out more about this mysterious Mr. Ferrel I asked "Where can I find this Perry Ferrel?"

With 'that' look in his eyes once again he stared at me saying "In my lab at the University's hospital. Are you able to stay in Heidelberg for another day? I would be most interested and happy to give you a tour of our facilities and we would be able to share even more ideas."

"Certainly I will stay for a couple of days." I responded.

"Good, then tomorrow you can go directly to the hospital and see Perry Ferrel. I will be busy until the afternoon. I will meet you in my lab and you and I can play around with Perry Ferrel to see what you think. Once you see Perry Ferrel I am sure that you will agree where we must go with our combined efforts."

"Very strange," I thought to myself, "who in the hell is this guy and why would I possibly want to 'play around' with him?" Very strange indeed I thought.

We reconvened after lunch and spent the rest of the day and evening fully engrossed, with the emphasis on *gross*, in the presentations and discussions of our colleagues. After the conference I simply returned to my hotel to digest the day's data as well as to try and fully decipher the previous day's notes. I ordered room service and retired early.

I awoke early and eagerly got showered and ready for my introduction to the very mysterious Mr. Ferrel. I still could not believe that I had not come across this guy in all of the years that I was in the business. How could I have missed him if he was so important? And my company, did they know anything about him? I decided to ask. I called the head of CT in Nurnberg and asked him if he had heard of this Perry Ferrel. He said that he had never heard the name before I had mentioned it but it sounded as if we would get along just fine as the name was American sounding. That was true. Now remember that Heidelberg is about 7 hours ahead of Philadelphia and it was 8:30 or so in Heidelberg. Not wanting to look too stupid or get caught off guard with the Ferrel guy I just had to do it, I had to call the American head of CT. Hey, if they did not want me to call them why would they have given me their personal phone numbers, right? I got a very groggy and somewhat disturbed "no" when I enquired about the mysterious Mr. Ferrel. I guess I was going to be on my own with this strange guy.

I made my way to the hospital and approached the information kiosk.
"Kann ich Ihnen helfen (can I help you)" the lady said.
"Sprechen Sie Englisch (do you speak English)?" was my slick reply.
"Yes I do," she politely said.
"I am here to see Mr. Ferrel," I said.
"Does he work here?"
"I really do not know whether he works here but Dr. Hilldenberg told me that he is here. He may be a visitor."
"Have a seat," she said, "I will try and find him."
After a few moments on the phone she asked,
"Would you know what department he would be with?"
"He should be in the cardiology department I would imagine," I said.
A couple more minutes passed and she slid the window open.
"No one in cardiology seems to know of Mr. Ferrel. Do you know his first name?"

"Perry," I said, "Perry Ferrel."
"Let me check our visitor log," she said.
A few more minutes passed.
"There is no one by that name registered in the log. Do you have an appointment with Dr. Hilldenberg?"
"Yes I do."
"Then sign the visitor log and I will give you a badge and directions to the cardiology department."
"Danke schön (thank you)" I said.
I went over and signed the book, got my badge and directions then headed for the Cardiology department.
The waiting room was packed; the sauerkraut and schnitzel thing no doubt. I walked to the reception window and asked if they spoke English. They did.
"I am here to see Mr. Ferrel, Perry Ferrel" I said.
"Is he a patient?" the lady asked in broken English.
"It is possible, but I really do not think so."
"Is he a doctor?"
"I really do not know that either, all I know is that Dr. Hilldenberg said that he would be here," I reluctantly said.
"Take a seat and I will see if I can locate Mr. Ferrel for you."
About five minutes passed and a man in the typical physician's cloak came out and said,
"Are you the one looking for Mr. Ferrel?"
"Yes" I replied.
"We had a call for him a few minutes back and we were unable to find him. He may be in the CT department."
He then turned around and left.
The lady was busy at the desk so I left the cardiology department to look for the CT department. I saw another smock-wearing lady walking down the hallway.
"Vo ist der CT-Abteilung (where is the CT department)?" I asked.
With a combination of gestures and very broken English she showed me where to go.

I entered the reception area and again asked for the elusive Mr. Ferrel. Another negative response. The girl said that she had never heard of a Perry Ferrel and she had been there for a few years. This was really getting weird. How could this Ferrel guy be that important and not one person, other than the good Dr. Hilldenberg, know who or where he was? "He may be out of the executive office on the 7th floor," she said. Why don't you check there?"

Up to the 7th floor I went. I got off of the elevator and went into the executive reception area. Again I managed to get a lady who could speak English. And once again I asked if she knew where I might find Mr. Ferrel. She said that she was not aware of anyone there by that name, however, the VP of clinical services was in and he had just had a conversation with a gentleman who had come in prior to her arrival and that she thought it may be Mr. Ferrel. She picked up the phone and talked for a moment to someone.
"What is your name?" she asked.
When I told her she repeated it to whoever was on the other end of the conversation.
And what company are you with?"
I told her and she again repeated it into the telephone.
"Mr. Ludwig our VP will be right out."
Before I knew it I was having coffee in the executive café with the VP who was quite inquisitive about my meeting with Dr. Hilldenberg and the elusive, mysterious Mr. Ferrel. All I could say was that it was regarding the future application of the technology.

Our impromptu meeting ended with Herr Ludwig telling me that he would try and locate Perry Ferrel and would report back to Dr. Hilldenberg. He reiterated his interest in the subject matter that would be discussed in such a meeting then sent me back down to the cardiology department.
It was early afternoon by then and I decided I would have lunch, relax a bit, take a stroll outside then meet with Dr. Hilldenberg in his lab. The introduction to this Perry Ferrel guy would have to wait until then... it's not like I didn't try, right?

At about 2:30 I made my way to the cardiac unit and then to the good doctor's office. He had just returned from his meetings.
"Kommen sie bitte in (come in please)" he said.
"Were you able to see Perry Ferrel?" he asked.

"No." was my reply.
"Why not?" he asked with 'that' look.
"I couldn't find him," I said.
"You couldn't find Perry Ferrel "he muttered as he sat down at his CT workstation.
"But Perry Ferrel is right here Herr Mueller."
Confused, I looked around and didn't see anyone else in the room but the two of us.
He quickly punched a few keys and his screen lit up.
"Here is Perry Ferrel," he said "here is the future of cardiovascular CT, here is Perry Ferrel."
As he spoke he pointed at the images on the screen, they were really neat showing the entire vascularity in the extremities, all of the peripheral vessels were there to be seen.

"Peripheral you idiot" I said to myself. "he was saying peripheral; not Perry Ferrel!"

Like I said, "I aint no cardiologist!"

Trust Me I Am Not A Doctor!

SECTION TWO

THE HUMAN ANATOMY

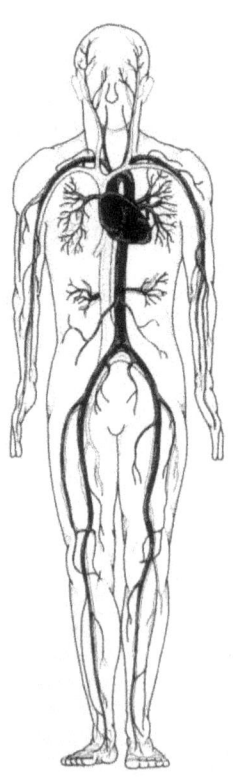

CHAPTER NINE
THE HUMAN HEART

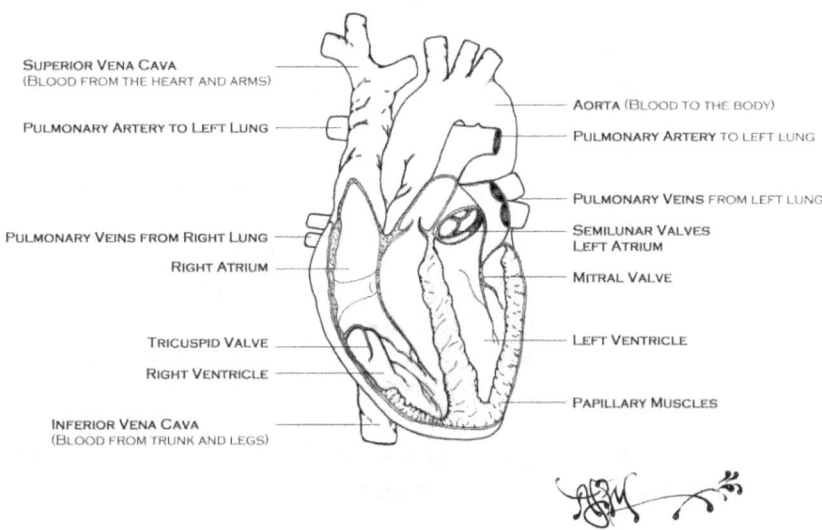

The heart, in the simplest of terms, is a pump. And like all pumps its function is to move fluid from one location to another. The fluid in this case is blood, and the locations are virtually every tissue and cell in the human anatomy. It is for this reason that the heart is unquestionably the most important of all organs in the body.

Situated in the middle of the chest cavity, the adult heart is a fist-sized bundle of muscle tissue held in place by a sac-like membrane called the pericardium and the connecting arteries and veins.

The heart contains two essentially identical, yet independent, systems consisting of an atrium, or upper chamber, and a ventricle, or lower chamber. As a result of their positioning, they are often referred to as the left heart and the right heart.

The pumping action of the heart is accomplished through a systematic cycle of rhythmic contractions and dilations or relaxations, of the heart muscle.

The contraction of the heart is referred to in medical terms as systole or the systolic cycle of the heart. The dilation, or relaxing action of the heart is called the diastole, or the diastolic cycle of the heart.

The actual rate of heart beat is in part controlled by the central nervous system which stimulates a special pacemaker in the right atrium near the superior vena cave.

This module then generates rhythmical pulses which travel along a bundle of neuromuscular fibers called the bundle of HIS, downward, branching off into two bundles.

Although these nerves influence the rate of heart beat, the heart muscle possesses the ability to induce contraction on its own and will continue beating at a regular rate even after complete separation from the nervous system.

Working like a double pump, one side of the heart pumps blood through the lung or pulmonary circuit, while the other side pumps blood to virtually all other parts of the body through a very complex system of arteries, capillaries and veins.

Veins bring blood back to the heart where it enters through the superior and inferior vena cava, the two large veins on the upper and lower right side of the heart. This blood collects in the right atrium, along with the blood which has been supplied to the heart muscle itself.

The blood is then drawn into the right ventricle following the beat. The heart then contracts and squeezes the blood into the pulmonary arteries and on into the capillaries of the lungs where the blood picks up oxygen.

The pulmonary capillaries then drain into the pulmonary veins, which brings this freshly oxygenated blood to the left atrium. This blood is then drawn into the left ventricle following a beat, after which contraction of the left ventricle rhythmically sends the blood into the aorta.

From the aorta, the blood is propelled to all arteries of the body, including the coronary arteries which furnish the heart muscle with fresh blood.

The blood expelled from one chamber during systole, or contraction, is refused re-entry during the diastole by four valves, called tricuspid and pulmonary on the right and mitral and aortic on the left.

The mitral and tricuspid valves separates the ventricles from the atria while the aortic and pulmonary separate the ventricles from the large arteries leaving the heart.

These valves sole purpose is to direct the flow of blood as well as prevent any backflow of blood to the heart.

The blood flows through the capillaries of the body tissue and into the veins returning to the heart through the superior and inferior vena cava, thus completing the cycle.

The healthy heart makes two distinct sounds during each cycle of the beat. The first being is a rather dull sound produced by the vibration and muscle fiber contraction which occurs at the same time as the valves which separate the atria from the ventricles close.

The second is very sharp and results from the rapid closing of valves which separate the ventricles from the aorta and the pulmonary arteries.

When heart disease occurs these sounds may be replaced or accompanied by murmurs resulting from damage or abnormal cardiac behavior, although murmurs may be heard in normal hearts. Detection of heart murmurs plays a most important role in the diagnosis of heart disorders.

CHAPTER TEN
THE HUMAN BLOOD

The main function of blood is to furnish the tissues of the body with a continuous supply of fresh oxygen, and to carry away the carbon dioxide wastes from these same tissues.

On the average, one eleventh of the total body weight of an individual is composed of blood. This is normally somewhere between 4.5 and 6 liters of blood.

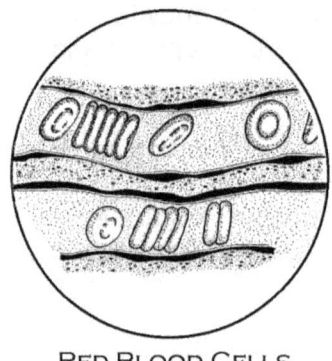 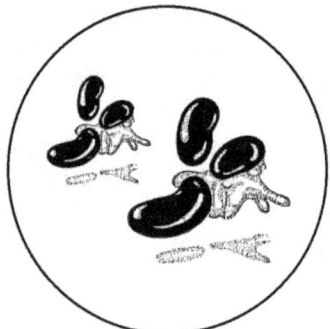

RED BLOOD CELLS (IN CAPILLARY)   BLOOD PLATELETS

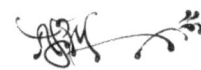

Blood is made up of four major components and these are:
- Plasma, a yellowish fluid whose main ingredient is water;
- Erythrocytes, or red blood cells;
- Leukocytes, or white blood cells; and
- Thrombocytes, or blood platelets.

Each of these components has a very specific and equally important function. Red blood cells, or Erythrocytes as they are properly called, contain compounds which readily combine with oxygen in the lungs and transport this oxygen to the tissues through which the blood passes. This oxygen is then released and replaced by carbon dioxide waste from these tissues which is taken back to the lungs for discharge through the breathing process.

White blood cells, or Leukocytes, are of two principal types both active in the battle against infection and disease. Certain white cells act in assuring immunity against certain diseases, while others release necessary substances to assist in the essential healing process after injury. White blood cells are the 'soldiers' of the system.

Plasma not only acts as the agent which allows blood to flow, but in itself contains components which function as carriers of essential tissue nutrients. Additionally, reactionary agents are contained in the plasma which themselves supply immunity against many diseases.

Blood platelets, or Thrombocytes as they are called, are suspended in the plasma and flow freely until injury occurs to the blood vessels. These platelets then adhere to the walls of the vessel at the point of defect, and plug it. The platelets then begin a disintegration process which in turn releases agents that assist in coagulation, the clot forming process, the very first step in the healing of any injury.

This 'clotting' ability of blood is one of its most remarkable properties. Clotting is essential in the healing process, yet sometimes this same miraculous ability, in itself constitutes a major threat to life! Blood clots sometimes form inappropriately. These clots then block the necessary passage of blood through the affected areas of the circulatory system resulting in heart attacks, strokes, and other dangerous and potentially fatal conditions.

Red blood cells (Erythrocytes), certain white blood cells (Leukocytes) and blood platelets (Thrombocytes) are all formed and continuously replenished by the bone marrow.

The specific white blood cells which have immunity functions are formed in the body's glandular system.

The components of plasma are formed in various assorted organs of the body.

CHAPTER ELEVEN
THE HUMAN LIVER

The liver is the largest of the internal organs of the body and is by far the most versatile. It acts as a chemical filter, stores vital nutrients, produces proteins and manufactures many other substances. Additionally, the liver breaks down many materials into more easily used components, and acts in a detoxification role.

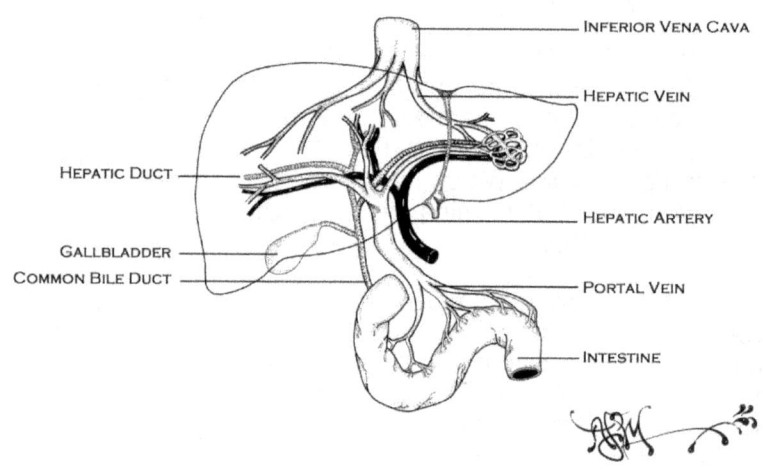

Located in front of the stomach in the upper right portion of the abdomen, this dark red, solid organ is unique in that, unlike any other organ, the liver has two sources of blood supply; the hepatic artery from the heart, and the portal vein from the stomach and intestines, through which it receives the nutrients supplied from the intestines.

These blood vessels penetrate the glandular tissue of the liver, and divide up into minute sinusoids, or microscopic divisions, between liver cells. Oxygen for the liver is received from the aorta by way of the hepatic artery.

Blood from the liver is drained into the hepatic vein, and it carries this blood to the inferior vena cava of the heart, where it will be pumped to the pulmonary, or lung circulation.

The liver is made up of minute divisions, known as lobules. These lobules consist of rows of cells surrounded by tiny channels referred to as canaliculi. Liver lobules are separated from each other by a connective tissue. These interconnected channels (canaliculi) collect the secretion of the liver, known as bile, and carry this bile to the hepatic duct. The hepatic duct joins the duct from the gallbladder, forming a common bile duct which empties into the duodenum, the first part of the small intestine.

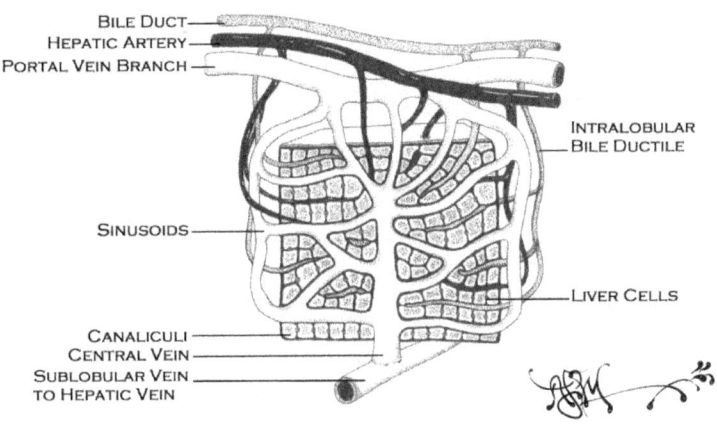

Blood flows through the liver at a rate of about 1.5 litres, or three pints, each minute. At any given time, the liver will contain about 10 per cent of the total blood supply of the body.

The liver helps the blood to assimilate food substances, as well as to detoxify waste materials, poisonous substances and to metabolize steroids and hormones. It stores sugars, minerals, vitamins and produces proteins, including many which act as agents in blood clotting, as well as in the production of the anti-coagulant heparin.

Nitrogen is removed in the liver and used to manufacture new protein from amino acids, using energy derived from carbohydrate or fat. The organ also produces fat, which it stores for later release to the body. The extraordinary activity of the liver generates a great amount of heat and, again, the liver shows its' versatility by playing a major role in the maintenance of proper body temperature.

CHAPTER TWELVE
THE HUMAN KIDNEYS

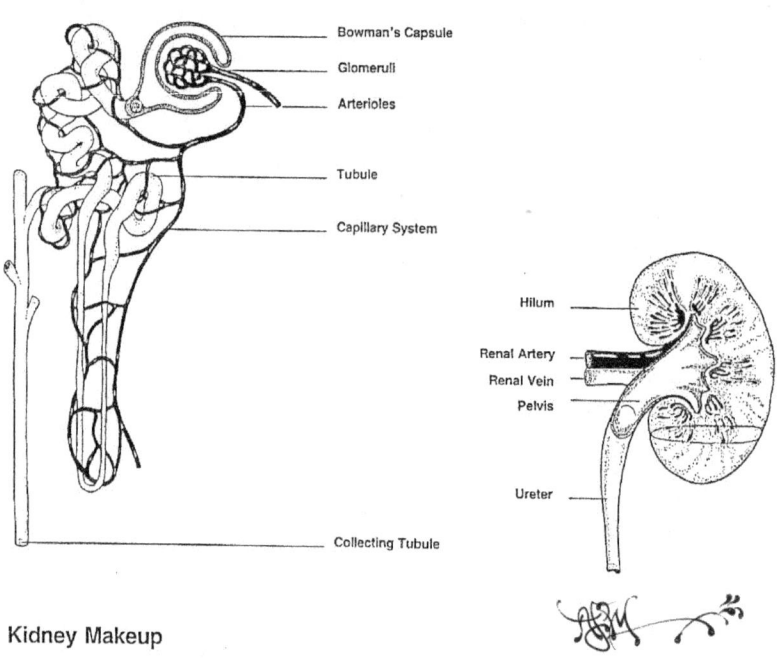

Kidney Makeup

Like most fluid systems, the body's cardiovascular circuit has a series of filters to extract certain substances and waste products from the blood.

One of the key filters in the anatomical system are the kidneys, a pair of organs whose function is to excrete urine containing waste products from the blood stream and to transport this urine to the bladder. The urine then is excreted from the body.

Human kidneys are located in the lower lumbar or loin region and rest on each side lateral to the spinal column. Surrounded by a heavy fatty tissue, these bean-shaped organs have a rounded outer border and a concave inner surface. The hilum, the indentation through which blood vessels enter and exit the kidneys, is on this inner surface.

The hilum arises from the kidney sinus, which is formed by the dilation of the ureter tube, forming a sac or kidney pelvis.

The kidney embodies a series of loops of capillaries called glomeruli, each situated in a thin envelope-like membrane called Bowman's capsules at the beginning of the renal tubules.

Blood enters the kidney through the renal artery and exits the kidney through the renal veins.

The blood flows through the capsules of the glomeruli, which filter out the water, salts and other waste products from the blood.

These extracted substances then flow down the renal tubules, which reabsorb some of the water and some salts. The remainder, along with additional secretions from the tubules, then makes the trip to the bladder and out of the body with the urine.

The average amount of urine secreted in a day is about 1.4 kilograms, or a little more than three pounds. This amount will vary with excessive perspiration or regurgitation (vomiting).

The kidneys act as a controller of fluid volume in the body, salt and acid concentrations.

The kidneys produce a hormone that assists in the production of red blood cells, or erythrocytes. They also excrete a hormone called renin, which assists the system to maintain proper levels of blood pressure.

Oddly enough, the kidneys are a key ingredient in the body's fight against high blood pressure, yet high blood pressure is a major contributing factor in renal failure, normally a fatal condition.

CHAPTER THIRTEEN
THE HUMAN SKIN

The skin is the largest organ of the body. It is the skin that provides the protective layer covering the external surface of the anatomy merging without any breaks with the mucous membranes of the internal canals at the orifices or openings in the body.

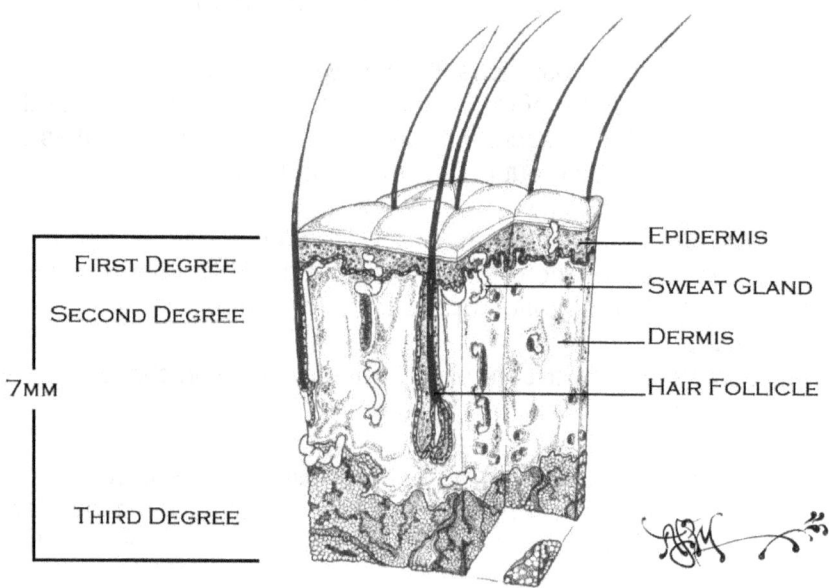

This covering forms a barrier against physical action, as well as against contamination of the deeper tissues from chemical and bacterial agents.

The skin, with very few exceptions (soles, palms, ears), is loosely attached to the underlying tissue and is elastic in nature.

The color of the skin under normal conditions is governed by the amount of pigment deposited in the skin cells from exposure to sunlight and differences in racial structuring.

Although the liver is the organ which regulates the chemical balances within the body, it is the skin that is responsible for the retention and exchanging of the vital fluid secretions which refresh and revitalize the entire body.

The skin is composed of two distinct layers: the epidermis or outer layer and the dermis or inside layer. The epidermis is without blood vessels and itself has two layers: and outer layer or crust of dead cells which are constantly worn away and replenished from below; and a sub-layer of germinating cells which become this upper layer.

The dermis or cutis vera (real skin) contains an elaborate network of blood vessels, nerves, sweat glands and hair follicles or roots. The subcutaneous layer of tissues below the dermis contains fat cells as well as blood vessels.

The interface of the dermis and the epidermis is very irregular with a series of fingerlike extensions varying length with the thickness of the skin. The ridged effect of the overlaying of these extensions in thick skin areas is what forms fingerprints and the other patterns on the palms and soles.

These extensions, or papillae as they are called, contain either loops of blood vessels or special nerve endings. These special nerve endings may be responsible for the sensation of touch.

Sweat glands or sudoriferous glands, as they are also known, are in all areas of the skin but are far more numerous and concentrated in the palm of the hands and the soles of the feet. These glands are small spiraling tubes which originate in the dermal layer and snake up extending through the epidermis. Sebaceous glands open into the hair follicles and secrete fatty matter which spreads upwards lubricating the skin.

Of all dangers which threaten the skin, burning is by far the most common. Without the proper function of the skin, the body loses its ability to control and exchange fluids, resulting in system failure and death.

Burns are classified in three major categories and these are:

First-degree burns in which only the outer or epidermal layer are minimally damaged which produces noticeable redness;

Second-degree burns which damage the epidermis

and extend into the bottom layer affecting the blood supply in limited areas. There is some transient formation of blisters to the top layer, but not usually causing scarring; and,

Third-degree burns destroy the skin organ in the affected area and terminate the blood supply to the burn area. Skin grafting or skin transplants are the only successful method to repair third-degree burns.

CHAPTER FOURTEEN
THE HUMAN EYE

The eye is among the smallest of the organs in the body, yet it is by far the most miraculous. The eye takes in simple light impulses and converts them into nerve patterns which allow for a neurological process that generates the beautiful colors and images that we see.

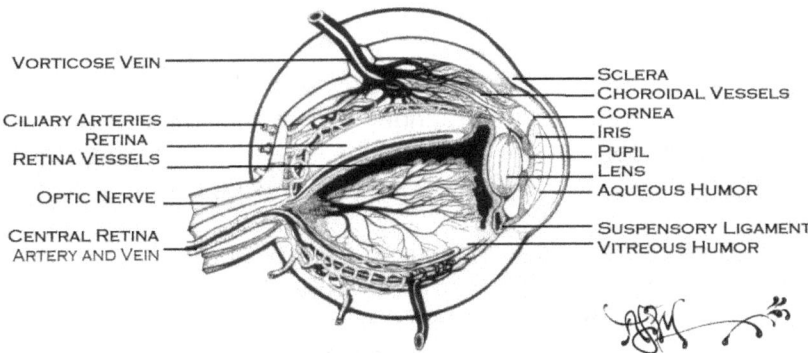

The human eyeball is spherical in shape, with a well pronounced bulge in the frontal area. Approximately one inch in diameter, its outer soft shell is composed of three distinct layers. The outside layer is referred to as the Sclera, the middle layer is the Choroid, and the innermost layer is the Retina.

The Sclera is a tough protective layer covering almost the entire eyeball and contains the transparent Cornea.
The Choroid, or middle layer of the eyeball, houses the Ciliary body of which the Lens is a part, as well as the Iris - the colored area in the central region of the front bulge of the eye.

The Retina is an extremely complex covering of lightly pigmented tissue on which rest light-sensitive receptor cells having conical and rod-like shapes. The central portion of the Retina is referred to as the Fovea Centralis - a yellowish colored spot directly behind the Pupil.

The Fovea Centralis is the area of greatest visual accuracy, and is made up of only the cone-shaped receptor cells. The retinal coating changes in structure as it spreads away from the Fovea Centralis by a systematic integration of the rod-shaped cells into the conical cells. The conical cells gradually decline in number until, at the perimeter of the Retina, only the rod-like receptor cells are present.

The Cornea is a five-layered membrane through which the electromagnetic vibrations of light pass, unrestricted, to the Lens which is located behind the Cornea.
The Lens is separated from the Cornea by a clear watery fluid called the Aqueous Humor.

The Lens is a flattened sphere of transparent fibers arranged in layers connected to, and surrounded by, muscle called the Ciliary muscle, which controls the shape of the lens and thus the distance the eye is focused to.

The colored Iris is located directly in front of the Lens, and has a circular opening in its center called the Pupil. The Iris is activated by a muscle which controls the size of the Pupil opening, thus controlling the amount of light entering in the main body of the eye.

The eyeball itself is kept extended by a sac-like membrane called the Hyaloid membrane which is filled to a positive pressure with a transparent, gelatinous fluid called the Vitreous Humor.

The eye functions in the following manner: The Retina picks up the electromagnetic vibrations of light from the objects in front of it. This light passes through the Cornea, through the Pupil and into the Lens where the image is inverted and projected onto the Retina. The retinal cells then convert these light signals to neural impulses which travel along the Optic Nerve to the Brain which generates the images which we see.

The cone-shaped cells are individually linked to other nerve fibers resulting in far greater neural stimuli by these cells, allowing for much more detailed images to be produced.
Rod-shaped cells, conversely, are joined together in clusters and respond to stimuli over a much wider area.

The focusing process of the eye, known as accommodation,

deteriorates with age causing a loss of focusing ability, or accommodation of the eyes, to closer working ranges.

The movement of each eyeball is controlled by six (6) eye muscles, and when functioning together, both eyes perform the task of converging, or focusing on a single point of observation, allowing for three-dimensional imaging, as well as judgments of distance.

The Eyelids, Eyelashes, Eyebrows, Tear glands, as well as the Orbit (the hollow openings in the skull where the eyes are set) are all protective devices for the eyes. Under normal conditions, human eyelids close by reflex approximately every six to seven seconds. If eye irritants are present, the eyelids will close at a more frequent rate and tears will be produced to flush away these foreign objects.

The eyelids contain a series of glands called Meibomian glands, which secrete a fatty matter which lubricates the eyelids as well as the lashes, to catch foreign objects and dust particles.

CHAPTER FIFTEEN
THE HUMN THROAT

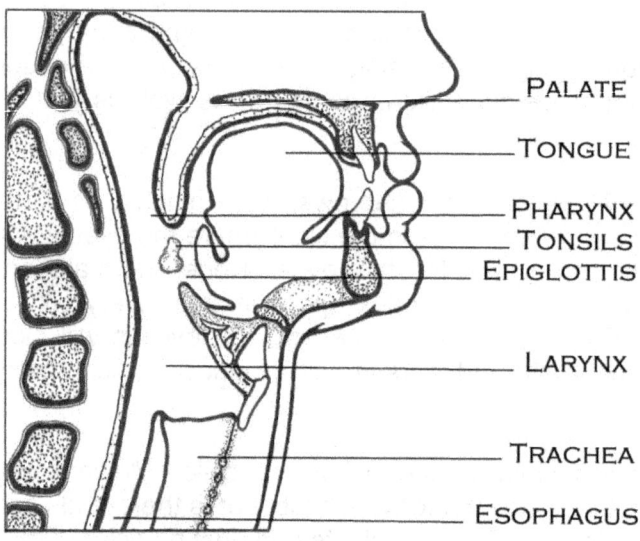

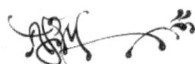

The human throat is a most complex structure of tissue, muscle, bone, cartilage and assorted organs. The throat is truly the body's lifeline for food and oxygen.

The throat provides a passageway from the mouth to the stomach through a canal-like tube called the esophagus.

It also provides a passageway for air from the nose and mouth to the lungs through the trachea or windpipe. The trachea carries the air we breathe that provides the lungs with continuous, fresh supply of essential oxygen. It also carries away carbon dioxide waste from the lungs.

The complexity of moving food from the mouth to the stomach is enormous and involves physiological harmony and complicated muscular control unmatched in any other bodily function. The average person will perform this neuro-mechanical miracle millions upon millions of times in his lifetime.

When one swallows, the entire throat mechanism is forced to make a most vital decision - which of the two passageways will be allowed to take in the food? Because of the restriction of space in the neck, the trachea and esophagus rest side by side. The opening for both rests just below the chin at the top of the neck, behind the Adam's apple or thyroid cartilage. When swallowing occurs, the thyroid cartilage rolls upward and stops for a moment. The food is then propelled to the back of the throat and into the esophagus, at which point, the cartilage drops back into place.

This simple action involves the neurological system that triggers the entire process and causes reflex contraction of the lips, jaws, tongue, throat and neck. The actual physical choice of sending the food down the esophagus is performed by the epiglottis, a leaf-shaped cartilage at the base of the tongue that covers the tracheal opening during swallowing.

All is well when this finely-tuned process works as planned, but like all complex systems, breakdowns do occur. Objects or liquids sometimes enter the wrong tube and cause respiratory system damage.

The most serious situation occurs when a morsel of food that is too large (generally more than 3.2 centimeters or 1" in diameter) settles over the opening of the trachea at the larynx. This causes choking. If the object does not dislodge itself, the vital oxygen supply is cut off.

The first system to be affected is the brain. There is panic, then blackout, then ultimately death if the obstruction is not removed.

The throat area also contains a series of lymph nodules embedded in and forming a ring around the back of the throat. These sac-like glands are filled with lymphoid tissues and function as protective devices for the pharynx or throat. These lump-like glands are known as tonsils.

Additionally, the throat plays a most vital role in the incredible ability of the human being to communicate with other humans. This capability centers around the voice box or larynx.

The larynx is an organ situated in the very uppermost part of the trachea or windpipe. This organ is a cartilaginous box containing two band-like membranes referred to as the vocal cords. These two cords, when their edges are drawn taut, vibrate in the passage of air from the lungs, producing sounds of variable pitch and tone.

The ability to control these sounds at will, or create speech, is what enables humans to vocalize with others, a very rare gift that separates humans from other creatures.

CHAPTER SIXTEEN
THE HUMAN EAR

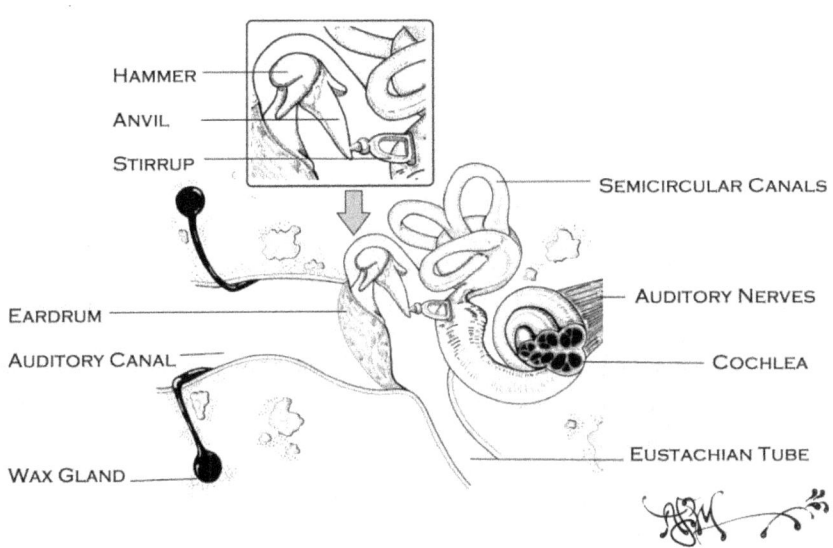

The ear is an organ with a double function. The first is to allow us to hear sound, while the second is less obvious, but equally important, giving us our sense of equilibrium or balance.

The ear is comprised of three distinct sections: the outer ear; the middle; and the inner ear.

The outer, or external ear, consists of the auricle or external flap of the ear, and of the auditory canal, a passage leading to the middle ear. This auditory canal is approximately three centimeters or 1 1/4 inches in length.

The middle ear is but a little over half an inch in length and contains the mechanism to conduct sound waves from the eardrum to the inner ear through a chain of three small bones called the ossicles. These bones are the malleus or hammer, the incus or anvil and the stapes or stirrup. The Eustachian tube, which connects the middle ear to the nose, permits entry of air into the middle ear.

The inner ear, or labyrinth, contains the actual organs of hearing and equilibrium that are connected directly to the auditory nerve. It is separated from the middle ear by the oval window. Part of the temporal bone, the inner ear, consists of the cochlea, the vestibule and three semi-circular canals. All of these membranous canals are filled with a fluid called endolymph.

The sensation of sound occurs when sound waves travel from the auditory canal to the eardrum. These waves cause a vibration of the eardrum which is transmitted by the ossicular bones through the oval window to the inner ear. The resultant movement of the endolymph (inner ear fluid) stimulates fine hair-like projections or ciliae in the cochlea. The deflection of these hair cells produce an electrical signal that is transmitted along the auditory nerve to the brain's auditory centers that perceive the sounds we hear. The semicircular canals and the vestibule also contain hair cells. These hair cells assist in responding to changes in the position of the head, a most important part of controlling equilibrium. The semicircular canals themselves provide sensory feedback on the movement of the head in all directions.

The eyes and tension on the body's muscles also assist in the maintenance of equilibrium, but when severe damage to the labyrinth occurs, problems of balance are inevitable. The brain, however, is able to compensate, so that within two to three months, one's balance is good enough to cope with most situations.

FINAL THOUGHTS
(at least for this book, I hope!)

My only real fear at this stage of my life as I finish this book is suffering a heart attack and waking up on the operating table with a rather agitated cardiologist wielding a scalpel staring down into my very blood-shot eyes who says "Mr. Mueller, I just read your book!"

How ironic would that be; I actually survive a massive heart attack but somehow I do not survive the cardiologist!

In the words of the immortal Alfred E. Newman *"what, me worry?"*

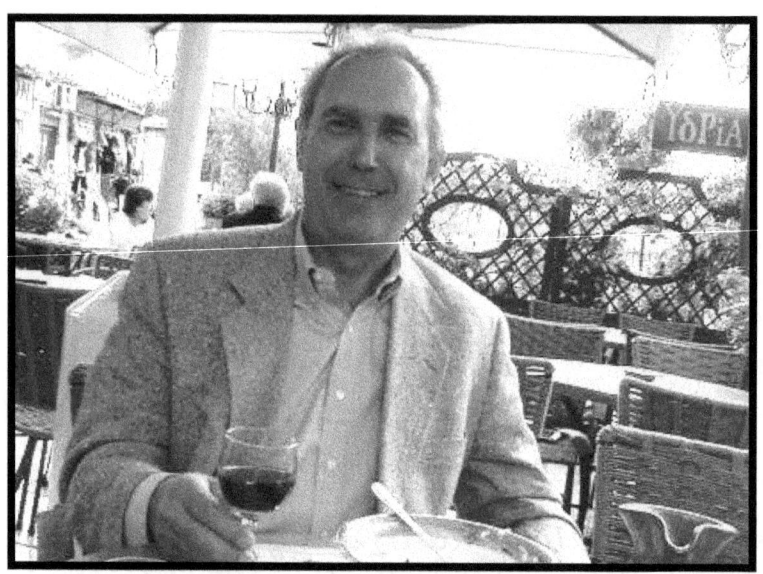

A.J. IN THE PLAKA AREA OF ATHENS, GREECE ENJOYING LIFE AND CONTEMPLATING THE MEANING OF THE PHRASE 'IT'S ALL GREEK TO ME'

ABOUT THE AUTHOR

A.J. MUELLER is a Cardiovascular Disease Management Consultant with International Cardiology Consultants and the National & International Heart Health Programs.

A.J. is also a freelance newspaper columnist, medical and technical illustrator, medical high-tech lecturer, former automobile and motorcycle racer, world traveler and general bon vivant. His present passions are medical technologies, classic automobiles, cooking and writing. He was born in Cincinnati, Ohio, raised in 'the Great White North, Canada, was a long-time resident of Florida and now resides in the very beautiful but very danger-laden Smoky Mountains of Western North Carolina.

A.J. can be reached at muellermedical@gmail.com

www.ingramcontent.com/pod-product-compliance
Lightning Source LLC
Chambersburg PA
CBHW071305040426
42444CB00009B/1882